Preface

Multiple choice questions are now used extensively in undergraduate and postgraduate examinations as an objective means of assessing students. They may also be used during and at the end of student courses to assess both learning and teaching.

Students often fear the Multiple Choice part of an examination because of the lack of familiarity and experience with this kind of assessment. The questions in this book are *not* intended primarily as examination practice, but rather for the student to assess his comprehension and learning of the obstetric and gynaecological course. The answer to virtually every question is to be found in the fifteenth editions of the companion books *Gynaecology by Ten Teachers* (**G**) and *Obstetrics by Ten Teachers* (**OB**) but not always on a single page!, although the occasional question may stretch the student's acquisition of knowledge a little further. The page references are to be found, for each question, on the answer page. The association with *Ten Teachers* does not preclude its usefulness to students who may wish to assess their knowledge from other textbooks and course material. At the same time, we hope it will help to familiarize students with MCQs and encourage them to pace themselves appropriately for examination conditions.

The subject of obstetrics and gynaecology remains part science and part art, and there are often opinions of various shades, making the setting of factual and objective questions particularly difficult.

We are grateful to the many colleagues who have offered constructive criticism of some of the questions, and to the authors of *Ten Teachers*, many of whom have contributed questions to this new Edition.

Acknowledgements

We thank our wives and families for their forbearance during many hours of preparation and discussion, and Mrs. M. Kates and Mrs. C. Whitehead for their careful typing of the manuscript.

M.E.S. London
R.J.L. Leeds
1991

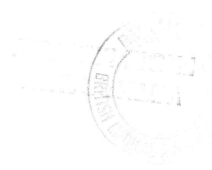

Gynaecology

1 The nerve supply to the vulva is derived from:
   (a) The pudendal nerve.
   (b) The ilio-inguinal nerve.
   (c) The genitofemoral nerve.
   (d) The posterior cutaneous nerve of the thigh.
   (e) The inferior haemorrhoidal nerve.

2 The support of the uterus is provided by:
   (a) The cardinal ligaments.
   (b) The round ligaments.
   (c) The utero-sacral ligaments.
   (d) The integrity of the perineal body.
   (e) The broad ligament.

3 Menstruation:
   (a) Is not normally accompanied by pain.
   (b) Contains blood, mucus and the unfertilized ovum.
   (c) The normal range of blood loss is 20–80ml.
   (d) Usually ceases before the age of 48.
   (e) Is often followed by fluid retention.

4 In the menstrual cycle, ovulation:
   (a) Occurs two days after the peak of LH.
   (b) Occurs 14 days before the onset of the menstrual flow.
   (c) Occurs when progesterone secretion is at its maximum.
   (d) Will only occur as a reflex response to orgasm.
   (e) May be inhibited by emotional disturbance.

5 After the menopause:
   (a) There is a reduction in vaginal acidity.
   (b) Gonadotrophin secretion falls.
   (c) Any vaginal bleeding should be investigated by performing a D. and C.
   (d) Treatment with oestrogen is often beneficial.
   (e) The rate of bone loss is greatest in the first two years.

6 Follicle-stimulating hormone (FSH)
   (a) Is responsible for Oestradiol production from the granulosa cells.
   (b) Brings about follicular rupture.
   (c) Is raised in polycystic ovary syndrome.
   (d) Is necessary for the initial stages of follicle development.
   (e) Is necessary for maintenance of the corpus luteum.

Multiple Choice Questions Gynaecology and Obs

with answers and explanatory comments.

Second edition

Marcus E. Setchell, MA, FRCS, FRCOG

Consultant, Department of Obstetrics and Gynaecology
St. Bartholomew's and Homerton Hospitals, London.

and

Richard J. Lilford, PhD, MRCP, MRCOG

Professor of Obstetrics and Gynaecology, St. James' Hospital, Leeds.

(Formerly Senior Lecturer, Queen Charlotte's Hospital, London).

Edward Arnold
A division of Hodder & Stoughton
LONDON MELBOURNE AUCKLAN

Contents

1 (a) **True**
  (b) **True**
  (c) **True**
  (d) **True**
  (e) **False**   This branch of the pudendal nerve supplies the anus and perianal skin.   **G 15/16**

2 (a) **True**
  (b) **False**   The round ligament may prevent retroversion, but does not support the uterus.
  (c) **True**
  (d) **False**   Unrepaired third degree tear does not lead to uterine prolapse.   **G 9, 10**
  (e) **False**   This is a peritoneal fold and contains no supportive tissue.

3 (a) **False**   Dysmenorrhoea may occur physiologically especially in young and nulliparous women.
  (b) **False**   The unfertilized ovum is autolysed in the fallopian tube some days prior to menstruation.   **G 23–25**
  (c) **True**
  (d) **False**   Fifty is the median age of the menopause.
  (e) **False**   Fluid retention precedes menstruation.

4 (a) **False**   Ovulation occurs about 32 hours after the onset of the LH surge (12 hours after the peak).
  (b) **True**   The length of the luteal phase is fairly constant, whilst the follicular phase may vary considerably.
  (c) **False**   Progesterone secretion increases very shortly before ovulation, reaching its peak in the mid-luteal phase.   **G 19–22**
  (d) **False**   In some animals coitus stimulates ovulation, but not in the human.
  (e) **True**   Pseudocyesis is a spectacular example, but other emotional phenomena may prevent ovulation.

5 (a) **True**   This may give rise to vaginitis.
  (b) **False**   There is an increase in FSH and LH production due to the loss of the oestrogen 'negative feed-back'.
  (c) **True**   It is essential to exclude carcinoma of the endometrium.   **G 31–33**
  (d) **True**
  (e) **True**

6 (a) **True**
  (b) **False**
  (c) **False**   LH is raised in the condition.
  (d) **False**   The *very* early stages of follicle development are hormone independent.
  (e) **False**   **G 26**

7 The occlusive diaphragm:
   (a) Should never be used for contraceptive purposes without contraceptive cream or jelly.
   (b) Should be used with at least two inches of contraceptive cream.
   (c) Should be left *in situ* for at least six hours after intercourse.
   (d) Is less reliable than the cervical (Dumas) cap.
   (e) May be particularly beneficial for prostitutes.

8 The combined oral contraceptive:
   (a) Predisposes to pelvic inflammatory disease.
   (b) Predisposes to benign breast and ovarian cysts.
   (c) Contains 0.2–0.5mg of ethinyl oestradiol.
   (d) May be less effective in patients with epilepsy.
   (e) Always contains 19 nor progesterone derivatives.

9 Intra-uterine contraceptive devices:
   (a) Should not be inserted at the time of suction termination of pregnancy.
   (b) Are radio-opaque.
   (c) Should be removed in early pregnancy if the threads are visible.
   (d) Should preferably be inserted at mid-cycle.
   (e) Are contra-indicated in patients with rheumatic heart disease.

10 The following are absolute contra-indications to use of the combined oral contraceptive:
   (a) Varicose veins.
   (b) A previous history of viral hepatitis.
   (c) A prosthetic heart valve.
   (d) Diabetes mellitus.
   (e) Carcinoma *in situ* of the cervix.

11 The following conditions are aggravated by the combined oral contraceptive:
   (a) Hirsuties.
   (b) Endometriosis.
   (c) Dysmenorrhoea.
   (d) Premenstrual tension.
   (e) Cervical erosion.

12 The risks of the intrauterine device in nulliparous women include:
   (a) Sterility.
   (b) Elevated serum copper levels.
   (c) Endometrial cancer.
   (d) Ectopic pregnancy.
   (e) Dyspareunia

7 (a) **True** The diaphragm by itself has little contraceptive effect and its function is to maintain a high concentration of spermicide at the cervical entrance.

  (b) **False** Four inches of cream is required.

  (c) **True** If intercourse is to take place repeatedly within this time it should be left for six hours after the last intercourse.

  (d) **False** **G 240**

  (e) **True** It protects against ascending infection and possibly to some extent against intra-epithelial neoplasia. It is less effective in this regard than the sheath which will also protect against herpes and AIDs (Acquired Immune Deficiency syndrome).

8 (a) **False** It may be protective.

  (b) **False** It protects against these conditions.

  (c) **False** It contains 20 to 50 micrograms, i.e. 0.02–0.05mg.

  (d) **True** Hydantoins and barbiturates potentiate hepatic conjugation and excretion. **G 234–237**

  (e) **False** Some new progestogens (e.g. gestodene) have been introduced.

9 (a) **False** There is no apparent increased morbidity with this practice.

  (b) **True**

  (c) **True**

  (d) **False** Shortly after menstruation is the recommended time. **G 238–240**

  (e) **True** Insertion predisposes to bacterial endocarditis.

10 (a) **False** Thrombo-embolism is not more likely unless the veins themselves are part of the post-thrombotic leg. **G 234–237**

  (b) **False**

  (c) **True**

  (d) **False** Insulin requirements may increase slightly but this is not an absolute contra-indication.

  (e) **False**

11 (a) **False** Suppression of gonadotrophins diminishes ovarian androgen production and this, together with the direct effect of oestrogen may, if anything, cause a slight and gradual improvement in hirsuties. **G 235–237**

  (b) **False** Oestrogens by themselves aggravate endometriosis but the combined pill causes shrinkage of normal and ectopic endometrium.

  (c) **False** ⎫
  (d) **False** ⎬ Elimination of ovulation usually improves these symptoms.

  (e) **True**

12 (a) **True** Because of ascending infection giving rise to salpingitis, which may be silent. **G 239–240**

  (b) **False**

  (c) **False**

  (d) **True** The risk is greater than with barrier methods or ovulation inhibitors. The risk per cycle is not increased in comparison with women using no contraception, but the cumulative risk is greater

  (e) **True**

13 Depo-provera:
   (a) Is usually used when contraception is required for more than two years.
   (b) Causes amenorrhoea in more than 50 per cent of cases.
   (c) Does not prevent conception after four months.
   (d) Should be given every three months.
   (e) Prevents endometrial hyperplasia.

14 Laparoscopic clip sterilization:
   (a) Can be reversed with greater success than vasectomy.
   (b) May be surgically reversed with better results than surgery, for post-infective tubal occlusion.
   (c) Is associated with a failure rate of one to two in 1000.
   (d) Has a higher failure rate when carried out at the time of termination of pregnancy.
   (e) Always requires general anaesthesia.

15 The following steroid structures are correct:

(a)

Oestrone

(b)

17α-Ethinyloestradiol

(c)

Diethylstilboestrol

(d)

17α-Hydroxyprogesterone

(e)

Testosterone

13 (a) **False**   It is licensed for short-term use only (although many authorities
                    consider it safe for longer term use)   **G 235**

  (b) **True**
  (c) **False**   Duration of action is variable after three months.
  (d) **True**
  (e) **True**

14 (a) **True**   Antisperm antibodies reduce the success of vasectomy rever-
                    sal.

  (b) **True**   Eighty per cent patency and 50 per cent pregnancy rates can be
                    expected after microscopic re-anastomosis and even better
                    results have been reported from selected centres. The outlook
                    for surgical repair after tubal diathermy is very poor.   **G 241**

  (c) **True**   Couples should be warned of this.
  (d) **True**
  (e) **False**   Local anaesthesia can be used.

15 (a) **False**   This is oestradiol.

  (b) **True**
  (c) **True**   **G 253–254**
  (d) **False**   The hydroxyl group should be in position 17, not 16 as shown
                    here.

  (e) **True**

16 Bromocriptine:
    (a) Is an analogue of prolactin.
    (b) Is used to treat hyperprolactinaemia.
    (c) Is a potent cause of multiple pregnancy.
    (d) May cause hypotension.
    (e) Effectively inhibits lactation after delivery.

17 The following hormones are active when given by mouth:
    (a) Oestradiol benzoate.
    (b) Equine conjugated oestrogens.
    (c) Ethinyloestradiol.
    (d) Norethisterone.
    (e) 17-Hydroxyprogesterone.

18 Therapeutic indications for progestogens include:
    (a) Endometriosis.
    (b) Fibroids.
    (c) Endometrial carcinoma.
    (d) Habitual abortion.
    (e) Dysfunctional uterine bleeding.

19 Luteinizing hormone-releasing hormone:
    (a) Stimulates release of FSH as well as LH.
    (b) Is a peptide of high molecular weight.
    (c) May be administered by single injection to stimulate ovulation.
    (d) Produces an exaggerated gonadotrophin response in hypogonadism.
    (e) Is produced by acidophilic cells of the anterior pituitary.

20 The following are indications for oestrogen treatment:
    (a) Fibroids.
    (b) Atrophic vulval dystrophy.
    (c) Post-menopausal vaginitis.
    (d) Threatened abortion.
    (e) Hypogonadotrophic hypogonadism.

21 The following hormones are predominantly oestrogens:
    (a) Dienoestrol.
    (b) Norethynodrel.
    (c) Premarin.
    (d) Androstenedione.
    (e) Norgestrel.

22 The following values of a semen analysis indicate *abnormal* semen quality:
    (a) Volume of less than 0.2ml.
    (b) Density of 40 million/ml.
    (c) Motility of 40 per cent.
    (d) Abnormal forms of 40 per cent.
    (e) Liquefaction complete in 30 minutes.

16 (a) **False**   It is a derivative of ergot alkaloid.
  (b) **True**
  (c) **False**   It is not associated with multiple ovulation.   **G 259**
  (d) **True**
  (e) **True**   Rebound lactation may however occur if it is stopped abruptly.

17 (a) **False**   Oestradiol valerate is orally active, and benzoate is used as an injectable preparation.
  (b) **True**
  (c) **True**   **G 253–258**
  (d) **True**
  (e) **False**   This is only active when given by intramuscular injection.

18 (a) **True**   Continuous administration suppresses cyclical bleeding from the endometrium, both normal and ectopic.
  (b) **False**   Fibroids may enlarge if progestogens are given.   **G 256–258**
  (c) **True**   Regression of metastases occur at least in a proportion of cases.
  (d) **False**   Although injections of progesterone have been widely used in the past for this purpose, there is no evidence of their efficacy.
  (e) **True**

19 (a) **True**
  (b) **False**   It is a low molecular weight decapeptide.
  (c) **False**   Its activity depends upon pulsatility, both physiologically and when used therapeutically. Continuous administration diminishes gonadotrophin secretion by down regulating its own receptor.   **G 259**
  (d) **True**
  (e) **False**   It is produced by neurosecretory cells in the hypothalamus.

20 (a) **False**   Indeed, oestrogens may accelerate the growth of fibroids.
  (b) **False**   Although this condition appears after the menopause, it does not respond to oestrogen treatment. Hydrocortisone and testosterone creams are used for symptomatic cases.
                                         G 254–256
  (c) **True**
  (d) **False**   The use of synthetic oestrogens in pregnancy predisposes the exposed female fetus to cervical and vaginal neoplasia in later life.
  (e) **True**   Puberty is induced with oestrogens and regular menstruation achieved with an oestrogen/progesterone preparation.

21 (a) **True**
  (b) **False**   This is a synthetic progestogen.   **G 253–256**
  (c) **True**   This is conjugated equine oestrogen.
  (d) **False**   This is a weak androgen.
  (e) **False**   This is a progestogen.

22 (a) **True**
  (b) **False**   The count is below 20 million to justify diagnosing oligospermia.
  (c) **True**   Motility should be at least 60 per cent.
  (d) **True**   Abnormal forms should be less than 30 per cent.   **G 225**
  (e) **False**   This is the normal liquefaction time.

23 Luteinising hormone releasing hormone (LHRH) Agonists:
    (a) Must be given by pump.
    (b) Cause initial gonadotrophin release.
    (c) Are effective in treatment of endometriosis.
    (d) Cause bone loss.
    (e) Relieve menopausal hot flushes.

24 The following are acceptable methods for confirmation of ovulation:
    (a) Basal body temperature drop at least 0.5° on the 14th day.
    (b) A day 21 blood progesterone level.
    (c) Histological examination of premenstrual endometrial biopsy.
    (d) Blood oestrogen level on the 13th day.
    (e) Demonstration of spinnbarkheit in cervical mucus.

25 Tubal patency may properly be demonstrated by:
    (a) Hysterosalpingography.
    (b) Air insufflation.
    (c) Laparoscopy and methylene blue dye insufflation.
    (d) Ultrasound.
    (e) Hysteroscopy.

26 The following are recognized complications of treatment of anovulatory infertility:
    (a) Multiple pregnancy.
    (b) Ectopic pregnancy.
    (c) Cervical mucus hostility.
    (d) Postural hypotension.
    (e) Ascites.

27 Clomiphene citrate:
    (a) Results in decreased cervical mucus production.
    (b) Blocks FSH release.
    (c) Results in increased LHRH release
    (d) Directly stimulates follicular growth
    (e) May result in ovarian hyperstimulation

28 In male factor infertility:
    (a) Men with hypogonadotrophic hypogonadism respond to Mesterolone (testosterone analogue)
    (b) Tamoxifen may increase spermatogenesis.
    (c) Steroids may decrease antisperm antibody levels
    (d) The post-coital test is usually positive
    (e) May be helped by GIFT

23 (a) **False**   LHRH itself is given by pump. The analogue (agonist) is given by nasal spray or injection.

(b) **True**   They are *agonists*. Commercially available antagonists are under development.   **G 259**

(c) **True**   With continued use they 'down-regulate' the pituitary. Endometriosis will usually recur when treatment is stopped.

(d) **True**   Due to hypoestrogenism.

(e) **False**   Flushes are a side-effect.

24 (a) **False**   A rise in temperature of 0.5° must be seen to be maintained over the last 14 days of the cycle.

(b) **True**

(c) **True**   Secretory changes in the endometrium only occur after ovulation.

(d) **False**   Oestrogen levels indicate follicular development, but not ovulation.   **G 226**

(e) **False**   This is a pre-ovulatory phenomenon dependent upon oestrogen.

25 (a) **True**

(b) **False**   Insufflation with CO_2 is acceptable, but with air there is a grave danger of air embolus.

(c) **True**   **G 226**

(d) **False**

(e) **False**   Hysteroscopy examines the uterine cavity, not the tubes.

26 (a) **True**

(b) **False**   Tubal surgery and *in vitro* fertilization may result in ectopic pregnancy but not ovulatory stimulation *per se*.

(c) **True**   Clomiphene, because of its anti-oestrogenic effect, may render cervical mucus hostile.   **G 228–229**

(d) **True**   This is a classical side-effect when bromocriptine treatment is started.

(e) **True**   Hyperstimulation with gonadotrophins may lead to ovarian cyst formation with ascites.

27 (a) **True**

(b) **False**   It is an anti-oestrogen which increases gonadotrophic production.   **G 228**

(c) **True**

(d) **False**

(e) **True**   The full-blown clinical syndrome is very rare with clomiphene used by itself.

28 (a) **False**   Gonadotrophins are necessary.

(b) **True**   But the fertility rate is not improved.

(c) **True**   **G 231**

(d) **False**

(e) **True**

29 In threatened abortion:
   (a) The uterine size is typically less than expected for the period of gestation.
   (b) Progesterone therapy is useful.
   (c) Pain is absent.
   (d) Vaginal bleeding is present in most cases.
   (e) Bed rest may prevent miscarriage.

30 Causes of first trimester abortion include:
   (a) Malaria infection.
   (b) Rubella.
   (c) Syphilis.
   (d) XO karyotype in the embryo.
   (e) Trisomy 21 in the embryo.

31 Septic abortion:
   (a) May result from exposure to gonorrhoea during pregnancy.
   (b) Is frequently due to a combination of coliforms and Bacteroides.
   (c) Is more likely to lead to septic shock than salpingitis or pelvic abscess in a non-pregnant patient.
   (d) Should be treated by immediate curettage of the uterus in all cases.
   (e) Is a less common cause of maternal death in Great Britain than it was twenty years ago.

32 In the diagnosis of ectopic pregnancy:
   (a) A ruptured corpus luteum cyst may cause identical clinical features.
   (b) Vaginal bleeding will be present in 99 per cent of all cases.
   (c) The standard pregnancy test is very useful.
   (d) Pain usually precedes vaginal bleeding.
   (e) A history of ten weeks amenorrhoea and pain in a patient who usually has 28 day cycles is highly suggestive.

33 Ectopic pregnancy:
   (a) Is associated with uterine enlargement.
   (b) Is situtated in the ovary in about 0.5% of all cases.
   (c) Is more dangerous when it is situated in the isthmus of the fallopian tube.
   (d) Can only be diagnosed after it has ruptured.
   (e) Is a complication of assisted conception.

29 (a) **False** This is a feature of missed abortion.
   (b) **False** Progesterone has been shown not to help and may interfere with external genital development in continuing pregnancies.
G 198–199

   (c) **True**
   (d) **False** Vaginal bleeding is *always* present, by definition.
   (e) **False**

30 (a) **True** Any high fever can cause abortion but malaria is particularly likely to do so because plasmodium parasitizes the chorio-decidual space. **G 196–197**

   (b) **True**
   (c) **False** The spirochaete does not cross the placenta until after 20 weeks of pregnancy.
   (d) **True** This is the commonest chromosomal abnormality in abortion material.
   (e) **True** Eighty per cent of 'Down's' embryos are aborted.

31 (a) **False** The cervical plug is a very effective barrier to ascending infection during pregnancy.
   (b) **True** **G 200–201**
   (c) **True** Pregnant patients are particularly predisposed to endotoxic shock.
   (d) **False** (i) Where bleeding is not heavy and the patient has a very high temperature, curettage should be deferred for six to 12 hours to give time for the antibiotic effect. Immediate surgical interference may lead to septic shock. Any pieces of infective material in the cervix should, however, be removed with sponge forceps. (ii) If the uterus is over 14 weeks in size, contractions should be induced by an oxytocin infusion.
   (e) **True**

32 (a) **True** This causes intraperitoneal haemorrhage (which is often considerable) after a short period of amenorrhoea. The differential diagnosis is not very important, however, as both conditions require laparotomy. **G 203–207**
   (b) **False** It is present in about 85 per cent of cases. It is often absent in those acute ectopics with intraperitoneal rupture of the isthmus.
   (c) **False** It is only positive in 50 per cent of cases; the more sensitive βHCG test may be useful.
   (d) **True** Pain usually comes first, in contrast with spontaneous abortion.
   (e) **False** Patients with ectopic pregnancy usually have a short history of amenorrhoea – six to eight weeks from the start of the last period. Ten weeks would suggest inevitable abortion.

33 (a) **True** Enlargement occurs due to growth of the myometrium under the influence of placental hormones. It is now, however, as large as a normal pregnancy of equivalent gestational age.
   (b) **True**
   (c) **True** This tends to lead to tubal rupture and massive intraperitoneal haemorrhage. Ampullary implantation more often leads to 'tubal abortion' with a more gradual accumulation of blood.
G 203–207
   (d) **False** Ultra-sound (especially transvaginal) can demonstrate an intact extra-uterine gestation, and this is used in high risk cases, e.g. previous ectopic pregnancy.
   (e) **True** There is a 3-fold increased incidence with IVF and GIFT.

34 Cervical incompetence:
    (a) Typically causes painful abortions.
    (b) Typically causes mid-trimester abortion.
    (c) Is treated by Shirodkar suture which is best performed early in the second trimester.
    (d) May be caused by hydramnios.
    (e) May lead to premature rupture of the membranes.

35 Complications of intra-uterine mid-trimester prostaglandin administration for termination of pregnancy include:
    (a) Disseminated intra-vascular coagulation (DIC).
    (b) Convulsions.
    (c) Utero-vaginal fistula.
    (d) Eclampsia.
    (e) Chorea gravidarum.

36 In the UK termination of pregnancy requires:
    (a) Consent from husband.
    (b) A surgical operation.
    (c) Consent from guardian of a minor.
    (d) Agreement of any two doctors.
    (e) Notification to the Department of Health

37 Pregnancy may be terminated using:
    (a) Prostaglandin inhibitors.
    (b) Progesterone inhibitors.
    (c) Suction evacuation.
    (d) Laminaria tents.
    (e) Beta blocking agents.

38 In Turner's Syndrome:
    (a) A chromosomal structure of 45 XY is characteristic.
    (b) Secondary amenorrhoea is usual.
    (c) Coarctation of the aorta may occur.
    (d) The ovaries are multicystic.
    (e) Pubic hair is absent.

39 Patients with the following conditions typically present with primary amenorrhoea:
    (a) Uterus didelphys.
    (b) Imperforate hymen.
    (c) Anorexia nervosa.
    (d) Testicular feminization.
    (e) Untreated congenital adrenal hyperplasia.

34 (a) **False**   The 'incompetent' cervix dilates easily; thus abortion is relatively pain-free in typical cases.

(b) **True**

(c) **True**   First trimester abortion for other reasons is common (15–20 per cent of all pregnancies); thus cerclage is best delayed until the second trimester. **G 197–198**

(d) **False**   Hydramnios, however, leads to premature delivery in its own right.

(e) **True**   The incompetent cervix typically presents with painless dilatation, followed by rupture of the membranes.

35 (a) **True**   This is caused by amniotic fluid embolus and is associated with DIC, shock lung and hypotension. **G 209–213**

(b) **False**   This can, however, result from water intoxication if oxytocin infusions are administered.

(c) **True**   Hypertonic uterine action after prostaglandin administration may lead to delivery through the posterior fornix.

(d) **False**

(e) **False**

36 (a) **False**

(b) **False**   Prostaglandins, anti-progesterones are but two of the pharmaceutical agents which may be used for termination.

G 209–213

(c) **True**

(d) **False**   Only *registered* medical practitioners who are not in partnership may sign the certificate (except in an emergency procedure when only one signature is required.

(e) **True**

37 (a) **False**

(b) **True**

(c) **True**   **G 209–213**

(d) **True**

(e) **False**

38 (a) **False**   45 XO is the commonest karyotype. Mosaics such as XO, XX may also occur.

(b) **False**   There is primary amenorrhoea.

(c) **True**   **G 49–50**

(d) **False**   The ovaries are streak-like structures.

(e) **True**

39 (a) **False**

(b) **True**   Strictly speaking this causes cryptomenorrhoea (i.e. retention of menstrual secretion) but it is a differential diagnosis of primary amenorrhoea. **G 49–55**

(c) **False**   This causes secondary amenorrhoea.

(d) **True**

(e) **True**

40 The following investigations may be relevant in cases of amenorrhoea:
    (a) Skull X-ray.
    (b) Pregnancy test.
    (c) Thyroid function tests.
    (d) Glucose tolerance test.
    (e) LHRH estimation.

41 In the polycystic ovary:
    (a) Obesity is common.
    (b) There is loss of body hair.
    (c) LH levels are low.
    (d) Irregular widely spaced menstruation is typical.
    (e) Clomiphene may restore ovulation and menstruation.

42 In testicular feminization:
    (a) The chromosome status is XXY.
    (b) The gonads should be removed after puberty.
    (c) The patient adopts a male role and appearance.
    (d) Breasts are absent.
    (e) The voice is female.

43 Post-coital bleeding may be a sign of:
    (a) Fibroids.
    (b) Adenomatous polyps.
    (c) Cervical erosion.
    (d) Dysplasia of the cervix.
    (e) Carcinoma *in situ*.

44 Heavy but regular periods are a likely feature of:
    (a) Fibroids.
    (b) Carcinoma of the cervix.
    (c) Dysfunctional uterine bleeding.
    (d) Myxoedema.
    (e) Hypertension.

45 Cystic glandular hyperplasia:
    (a) Is associated with low oestrogen levels.
    (b) May predispose to endometrial carcinoma.
    (c) Is caused by a virus transmitted in cheese.
    (d) Occurs with ovulatory failure.
    (e) Generally occurs post-menopausally.

40 (a) **True**   This is often done to visualize the pituitary fossa.
   (b) **True**   One must never overlook the possibility of pregnancy.
                                                              G 172–173
   (c) **True**   Both myxoedema and hyperthyroidism may cause amenorrhoea.
   (d) **False**   Although severe diabetes may cause amenorrhoea, it is unlikely
to be a presenting symptom.
   (e) **False**   LHRH stimulation tests are sometimes carried out, but LHRH
assay is not routinely available.

41 (a) **True**
   (b) **False**   There is usually hirsuties.
   (c) **False**   There is a relatively high LH level compared with FSH.   **G 170**
   (d) **True**
   (e) **True**

42 (a) **False**   Chromosome karyotype is XY.
   (b) **True**   There is a five per cent risk of development of dysgerminoma.
   (c) **False**   They are invariably female in appearance.   **G 50**
   (d) **False**   The breasts are fairly well developed after puberty.
   (e) **True**

43 (a) **True**   From a fibroid polyp.
   (b) **True**   This benign endometrial polyp may, rarely, extrude through the
cervix.
   (c) **True**   **G 179**
   (d) **False**
   (e) **False**

44 (a) **True**
   (b) **False**   This usually causes irregular bleeding.
   (c) **True**   The ovulatory forms of dysfunctional uterine bleeding are often
regular. Anovulatory dysfunctional bleeding seen with severe
polycystic ovary syndrome and at the extremes of reproductive
life is irregular.   **G 174–178**
   (d) **True**
   (e) **False**

45 (a) **False**   In the early phase of the menopause, oestrogen levels are maintained, but ovulation does not occur. This leads to a thickened
cystic endometrium which sheds irregularly. Lack of progesterone means that the normal tortuosity and constrictor effect
on spiral arterioles is lost.   **G 176–177**
   (b) **True**   The endometrial hyperplasia may be atypical with danger of
progression to carcinoma.
   (c) **False**
   (d) **True**
   (e) **False**   It occurs in puberty and peri-menopausally.

46 Premenstrual tension syndrome:
  (a) Mostly occurs in women under 25.
  (b) Is often accompanied by depression and irritability.
  (c) Is only relieved when the menstrual flow is completed.
  (d) Is exacerbated by psycho-social factors.
  (e) May be associated with acts of crime.

47 Effective treatments for primary (spasmodic) dysmenorrhoea include:
  (a) Diuretics.
  (b) Flufenamic acid.
  (c) Fenfluramine.
  (d) Combined contraceptive pills.
  (e) Pre-sacral neurectomy.

48 Candida infection has a recognised association with:
  (a) Oral contraception.
  (b) Chronic renal disease.
  (c) Antibiotic treatment.
  (d) The menopause.
  (e) Cervical dysplasia

49 The following organisms are known causes of pelvic inflammatory disease:
  (a) Stretpococcus pyogenes.
  (b) Herpes simplex.
  (c) Chlamydia.
  (d) Clostridium welchii.
  (e) Trichomonas.

50 Tuberculosis of the female genital tract:
  (a) Most commonly affects the fallopian tubes.
  (b) Is usually sexually transmitted.
  (c) May cause ascites.
  (d) Causes infertility.
  (e) Is best diagnosed by taking an endometrial biopsy in the first half of the
    cycle.

51 In women with syphillis:
  (a) The incubation may be as long as three months.
  (b) A chancre will be seen in most cases.
  (c) If the VDRL is positive, the TPHA will be negative.
  (d) General paralysis of the insane may result.
  (e) Tetracyclines may be used for treatment.

52 Chlamydial infection is:
  (a) The most common cause of STD.
  (b) Caused by an intracellular organism.
  (c) Silent in over half of cases.
  (d) Sensitive to metronidazole.
  (e) A possible cause of pneumonia in infants.

46 (a) **False** It is commoner in women over 30.
   (b) **True**
   (c) **False** It is usually relieved by the *start* of the menstrual flow.
   (d) **True**   **G 181**
   (e) **True** There is an increased incidence of shop-lifting, etc., and even major acts of violence are said to occur more often in the pre-menstrual phase.

47 (a) **False**
   (b) **True**
   (c) **False** This agent is an appetite suppressant.   **G 179–180**
   (d) **True**
   (e) **True** This operation is not often performed now, as simpler treatments are usually effective.

48 (a) **True**
   (b) **False**
   (c) **True**
   (d) **False**   **G 75–77**
   (e) **False** This is in contrast to the typical sexually transmitted infections such as trichomonas and papilloma virus.

49 (a) **True** The organism is often responsible for post-abortion or post-delivery infection.
   (b) **False**   **G 82–87**
   (c) **True** This and Neiserria gonococci cause more than two thirds of cases, but super-infection with other organisms usually occurs.
   (d) **True** May occur following criminal abortion.
   (d) **False** Affects the vagina only.

50 (a) **True**
   (b) **False** It is nearly always secondary to pulmonary tuberculosis.
   (c) **True**   **G 87–90**
   (d) **True** The tubes are almost invariably infected and even after full chemotherapy, restoration of fertility is unusual.
   (e) **False** It is necessary to take a biopsy in the second half of the cycle when the granulomata have had time to develop.

51 (a) **True**
   (b) **False** Women usually present with secondary disease because the chancre is not noticed as it is not exposed.   **G 99–100**
   (c) **False** The VDRL is based on IgM and becomes negative more rapidly after successful treatment.
   (d) **True**
   (e) **True**

52 (a) **True**
   (b) **True**
   (c) **True**   **G 97**
   (d) **False**
   (e) **True**

53 HIV Carriers:
   (a) Are always serum antibody positive.
   (b) Have a better prognosis with treatment.
   (c) Cannot transmit the disease until they develop the clinical syndrome.
   (d) Transmit the virus to the fetus in over 80 per cent of cases.
   (e) Will almost certainly not develop the disease.

54 Gonorrhoea:
   (a) Infects the vaginal epithelium.
   (b) May cause arthritis.
   (c) May be symptomless.
   (d) Is diagnosed by a serological test.
   (e) Crosses the placenta.

55 Tubal disease is a recognised complication of:
   (a) Asymptomatic chlamydial salpingitis.
   (b) Pneumococcal salpingitis.
   (c) Intrauterine devices.
   (d) Ovarian cystectomy.
   (e) Actinomycosis.

56 Acceptable treatment for Uterine fibroids includes:
   (a) No treatment.
   (b) Myomectomy during pregnancy if red degeneration occurs.
   (c) Cyclical oestrogen treatment.
   (d) Vaginal myomectomy.
   (e) Caesarean hysterectomy.

57 Fibroids:
   (a) May protrude through the cervix.
   (b) Are composed mostly of fibrous tissue.
   (c) Are more common in infertile patients.
   (d) Are rare in negresses.
   (e) Commonly arise from the cervix.

58 Complications of fibroids include:
   (a) Intraperitoneal haemorrhage.
   (b) Endometrial carcinoma.
   (c) Obstructed labour.
   (d) Polycythaemia.
   (e) Recurrent abortion.

59 Endometriosis is a recognised cause of:
   (a) Deep dyspareunia.
   (b) Amenorrhoea.
   (c) Dysmenorrhoea.
   (d) Post-menopausal bleeding.
   (e) Painful laparotomy scar.

53 (a) **False** Most cases develop antibodies within three months of infection.
   (b) **True**
   (c) **False**   **G 101–105**
   (d) **False** Transplacental spread occurs in less than half of cases.
   (e) **False**

54 (a) **False** It infects glandular epithelium such as the cervix or urethra.
   (b) **True**
   (c) **True**   **G 97–98**
   (d) **False** The gonoccocal complement fixation test is notoriously un-reliable and does not become positive until some weeks after infection.
   (e) **False** Gonoccocal ophthalmia may be acquired by the baby during delivery, but the organism does not cross the placenta.

55 (a) **True**
   (b) **False**
   (c) **True** Ascending pelvic infections are more common especially in nulliparous women.   **G 83–87**
   (d) **True** The fimbriae may become involved in peritubal adhesions.
   (e) **True**

56 (a) **True** If tumours are small (!ess than the size of a 12 week pregnancy) and asymptomatic, this is the appropriate management.
   (b) **False** This can be highly dangerous, causing severe haemorrhage, and is likely to initiate labour.   **G 110–119**
   (c) **False** This tends to cause enlargement of fibroids.
   (d) **True** This is appropriate for pedunculated submucous fibroids.
   (e) **True** If no further pregnancies are desired.

57 (a) **True** Submucosal fibroids may become polypoid and be extruded through the cervix where they ulcerate and become infected.
   (b) **False** They are composed mostly of smooth muscle.   **G 110–119**
   (c) **True** They are more common in people who are subfertile and, once formed, they may contribute further to subfertility.
   (d) **False** They are three times more common than in caucasians.
   (e) **False** Only two per cent arise in this site.

58 (a) **True** From rupture of a surface vessel.
   (b) **False** Sarcoma is found in 0.2 per cent.   **G 110–119**
   (c) **True**
   (d) **True** This is probably due to erythropoetin secretion by the tumour.
   (e) **True**

59 (a) **True** This is one of the classical features along with dysmenorrhoea, Pain and menorrhagia.
   (b) **False** Significant hormone imbalance is not a feature.   **G 164–167**
   (c) **True**
   (d) **False**
   (e) **True** Rarely, ectopic endometrium may appear in scars.

60 Endometriosis:
   (a) Is the commonest cause of chronic lower abdominal pain in young women.
   (b) Most frequently involves the ovaries.
   (c) Often flares up during pregnancy.
   (d) Is associated with subfertility.
   (e) Is more common in Negro races.

61 The following are useful for the treatment of endometriosis:
   (a) Danazol.
   (b) Duphaston.
   (c) LHRH analogues.
   (d) The oral contraceptive.
   (e) Prednisolone.

62 The following vulval conditions cause pruritus vulvae:
   (a) Hypertrophic dystrophy.
   (b) Lymphogranuloma venereum.
   (c) Condylomata acuminata.
   (d) Syphilitic chancre.
   (e) Threadworms.

63 The vulva:
   (a) May be the site of primary trichomonas infection
   (b) Is the site of five per cent of all malignant growths of the female reproductive tract.
   (c) Becomes atrophic after the menopause.
   (d) May be the site for lichen sclerosis et atrophicus.
   (e) May be involved in primary, secondary and tertiary syphilis.

64 Bartholin's cysts:
   (a) Should always be excised to prevent recurrence.
   (b) Are situated on the inner side of the posterior end of the labium majus.
   (c) May become infected by gonorrhoea.
   (d) Are usually bilateral.
   (e) May be easily confused with hidradenoma.

65 Carcinoma of the vulva:
   (a) Does not ulcerate until it is is advanced.
   (b) Is usually histologically anaplastic.
   (c) Spreads initially to iliac nodes via vaginal lymphatics.
   (d) Seldom involves lymph nodes at the time of presentation.
   (e) Is equally amenable to treatment by surgery and radiotherapy.

66 Cervical smears:
   (a) Are taken with a throat swab.
   (b) Should be placed in fixative immediately.
   (c) Should be taken every ten years.
   (d) Are negative in up to 100% of cases of established cervical cancer.
   (e) Should not be done in women under 21.

60 (a) **False** In most cases of chronic pelvic pain, no cause is found.
   (b) **True** The peritoneum of the broad ligament and Pouch of Douglas is the second commonest site. **G 164–167**
   (c) **False** The disease regresses during pregnancy.
   (d) **True**
   (e) **False** Fibroids are more common in the Negro race; endometriosis in Caucasians.

61 (a) **True**
   (b) **True**
   (c) **True**
   (d) **True** The beneficial effect is due to the progestogen.
   (e) **False** **G 167–168**

62 (a) **True**
   (b) **False** The ulcers are characteristically painless.
   (c) **True** Vulval warts may be intensely itchy.
   (d) **False** Chancre is classically painless and non-irritant. **G 71–75**
   (e) **True** In children the migration of anal threadworms may cause vulval irritation.

63 (a) **False**
   (b) **True**
   (c) **True** **G 71–75**
   (d) **True**
   (e) **True** Gumma formation may occur in tertiary syphilis, condylomata lata in secondary disease and chancre in primary syphilis.

64 (a) **False** Marsupialization is the primary treatment of choice as it it a smaller operation and preserves the function of the gland. **G 106**
   (b) **True**
   (c) **True**
   (d) **False**
   (e) **False** Hidradenoma is a small (less than 2cm), solid benign tumour of sweat glands.

65 (a) **False** Ulceration is usually an early sign.
   (b) **False** It is usually well differentiated. **G 107–108**
   (c) **False** Spread is to the inguinal nodes.
   (d) **False** These lymph nodes are involved in 50 per cent of cases at presentation.
   (e) **False** Surrounding tissues will not tolerate effective doses of radiotherapy.

66 (a) **False** An Ayre's spatula is used.
   (b) **True** Air drying spoils the preparation. **G 122–124**
   (c) **False** A smear should be repeated every three years ideally.
   (d) **True**
   (e) **False** All sexually active women should have smears done regularly.

67 Carcinoma *in situ* of the cervix:
   (a) Arises from the squamo-columnar junction.
   (b) Usually becomes invasive within three to four years.
   (c) Causes a 'mosaic' appearance on colposcopy.
   (d) May regress spontaneously.
   (e) Merges gradually with healthy epithelium.

68 Cone biopsy of the cervix:
   (a) Should be carried out on all patients with carcinoma *in situ* unless hysterectomy is required for some other reason.
   (b) May cause secondary haemorrhage, with a peak incidence 14–21 days after the operation.
   (c) Has been carried out more frequently since the discovery of colposcopy.
   (d) Is required for symptomatic cervical erosions.
   (e) Increases the chances of caesarean section in a subsequent pregnancy.

69 Endocervical carcinoma:
   (a) Is usually an adenocarcinoma.
   (b) May spread directly to para-aortic nodes.
   (c) Usually causes death from local invasion before metastases become manifest.
   (d) Causes a barrel shaped cervix.
   (e) Is usually diagnosed by means of a cone biopsy.

70 Stage I cancer of the cervix:
   (a) Is confined to the uterus.
   (b) May not be visible on clinical examination.
   (c) Has a better prognosis than Stage I cancer of the endometrium.
   (d) May be associated with hydro-ureter on intravenous pyelogram.
   (e) May be treated with intracavity radiation (to provide 7 000 rads at point A) and external radiotherapy.

71 Radiotherapy for carcinoma of the cervix may cause:
   (a) Vesico-vaginal fistula.
   (b) Pyometra.
   (c) Proctitis.
   (d) Acute salpingitis.
   (e) Ovarian failure.

67 (a) **True**
   (b) **False**   Ten years is the mean time for invasive change.
   (c) **True**   **G 121–122**
   (d) **True**
   (e) **False**   The junction between healthy and abnormal epithelium is abrupt.

68 (a) **False**   Laser treatment, coagulation or some other form of 'ablation' may be employed, provided the whole ectocervix can be inspected through the colposcope.   **G 128–129**
   (b) **False**   The peak incidence for secondary haemorrhage is seven to ten days postoperatively.
   (c) **False**   Colposcopy allows selective biopsy of the affected areas to be carried out and ablation employed if no invasion is detected. Cone biopsy can therefore be reserved for those cases where the squamo-columnar junction is high in the endocervical canal and cannot be visualized through the colposcope.
   (d) **False**   These are treated by cryosurgery or coagulation.
   (e) **True**   Cervical stenosis (fibrosis) may prevent dilatation, although no difficulty is experienced in the majority of cases.

69 (a) **False**   Squamous metaplasia usually precedes malignancy.
   (b) **True**   In this case, spread occurs along the ovarian lymphatics.
                                                      G 129
   (c) **True**   As with ectocervical cancer, renal failure (due to ureteric obstruction) is the commonest cause of death.
   (d) **True**
   (e) **False**   This is used for carcinoma *in situ* and dysplasia when an adequate colposcopically-directed biopsy is impossible, most often because the squamo-columnar junction cannot be seen.

70 (a) **True**
   (b) **True**   This is Stage Ia.
   (c) **False**   Spread to lymph nodes is more common. The five-year corrected survival rates are 75 per cent for Stage I cancer of the cervix, and 90 per cent for endometrial cancer.   **G 132–133**
   (d) **False**   This would be classified as Stage III, as staging takes into account normal pre-operative investigations.
   (e) **True**   Radiation dose diminishes by the inverse square law and therefore separate internal and external doses are required to cover local lesion and pelvic nodes.

71 (a) **True**   But this is very rare with modern treatment in the absence of a recurrence. However, if tumour has eroded the bladder prior to treatment, this is more likely.   **G 133–134**
   (b) **True**   Secretions may accumulate behind a fibrotic and stenosed cervix.
   (c) **True**   This is the most common side-effect. It is treated with steroid suppositories.
   (d) **False**
   (e) **True**   This is inevitable.

72 Carcinoma of the endometrium:
  (a) Is very rare (less than 5%) before the menopause.
  (b) Is more common in postmenopausal women on combined oestrogen, progesterone preparations.
  (c) Is usually (over 50%) a squamous carcinoma.
  (d) Is best treated by simple hysterectomy with conservation of the ovaries in early cases.
  (e) May be diagnosed by cervical cytology in 25–30% of cases.

73 Stage 1 carcinoma of the endometrium:
  (a) Is best managed by vaginal hysterectomy.
  (b) Is confined to the uterus.
  (c) Will have spread to lymph nodes in approximately ten per cent of patients.
  (d) Is the commonest stage at the time of diagnosis.
  (e) Should be treated with post operative radiotherapy.

74 Radiotherapy for cancer of the cervix:
  (a) May be curative.
  (b) Has approximately the same success rate as Wertheim's hysterectomy for Stage I lesions of the ectocervix.
  (c) Should not be used after a Wertheim's hysterectomy.
  (d) May consist of two intracavity caesium applications followed by external irradiation to the pelvic side walls.
  (e) Can be repeated if the tumour recurs after the initial standard dose (5 000–8 000 cGy)

75 Curative radiotherapy for gynaecological malignancy:
  (a) Is dependent mainly on beta rays.
  (b) May consist of intracavity radium or caesium and external radiation from supervoltage X-ray machines or cobalt.
  (c) May involve intracavity cobalt.
  (d) May be repeated after two years for a local recurrence.
  (e) Is potentiated by hypoxia.

76 Incontinence of urine:
  (a) Is commonly caused by prolapse.
  (b) May be caused by diabetes mellitus.
  (c) May be due to overflow incontinence in multiple sclerosis.
  (d) May be congenital.
  (e) Is best treated surgically if detrusor instability is the cause.

72 (a) **False** Although the peak incidence is between the ages of 50 and 65, 20–25% of cases occur premenopausally.

(b) **False** Unopposed natural (from granulosa cell tumours, polycystic ovary syndrome) or exogenous oestrogen predisposes to cancer of the endometrium; combined therapy does not. Indeed, there is now evidence that it is protective against this disease.

G 136–138

(c) **False** It is usually adenocarcinoma, or occasionally, a mixture of adeno and squamous.

(d) **False** The ovaries are a common site for metastases and oestrogen secretion activates any residual cancer cells.

(e) **True**

73 (a) **False** This procedure should only be used if the patient is a very poor operative risk and it is usually followed by radiotherapy.

(b) **False** It is confined to the *body* of the uterus. If the cervix is involved, it is classed as Stage II. This is in contrast to cancer of the cervix which is Stage I provided it is confined to the uterus as a whole.

G 138–139

(c) **True**

(d) **True** Eighty per cent of cases are Stage I.

(e) **False** Only cases with poor prognostic features such as deep myometrial invasion or poor differentiation should be treated in this way.

74 (a) **True** For example, 80–90% of Stage I ectocervical cancers can be cured by this treatment.

(b) **True** This has been confirmed by several large series.

(c) **False** If cancerous lymph nodes are removed, irradiation to the pelvic side-walls is often used. **G 133–134**

(d) **True** This is the widely used Manchester technique for cancer of the cervix.

(e) **False** The maximum dose of radiation which tissues will tolerate is 8000 cGy which cannot be repeated.

75 (a) **False** It is dependent on gamma rays; beta rays (electrons or positrons) and alpha particles are screened out.

(b) **True** **G 133–134**

(c) **True** Cobalt is usually used for external irradiation, but a machine known as the cathetron can be used to administer intracavity cobalt irradiation.

(d) **False** This has a high risk of causing extensive necrosis and fistula formation.

(e) **False** The reverse is true.

76 (a) **False** It is associated with, but not caused by prolapse.

(b) **True** Diabetic neuropathy may lead to *overflow* incontinence, as with other lower motor neurone lesions. **G 247–250**

(c) **False** This causes high pressure, urge incontinence as with other upper motor neurone lesions.

(d) **True** Occasionally a ureter may drain directly into the vagina.

(e) **False** Surgery is reserved for genuine stress incontinence.

77 Stress incontinence of urine:
    (a) Is more common in multiparous patients.
    (b) Can be controlled by para-urethral pressure during vaginal examination.
    (c) Can be diffentiated from urge incontinence by means of a cystometro-
        gram.
    (d) Should be investigated by cystoscopy prior to surgery.
    (e) May be a transient problem after delivery.

78 Uterovaginal prolapse:
    (a) Is a very painful condition.
    (b) The condition is worse in the erect position.
    (c) The cervix is often elongated.
    (d) Is common in Negroes.
    (e) May cause intestinal obstruction if there is a large rectocele.

79 Retroversion of the uterus:
    (a) Occurs in 15% of normal women.
    (b) Is a common cause of infertility.
    (c) May be corrected by a Fothergill operation.
    (d) Is caused by heavy lifting.
    (e) Should always be corrected with a Hodge pessary in early pregnancy.

80 Cystocele:
    (a) Is a prolapse of the bladder and anterior vaginal wall.
    (b) Is common after the menopause.
    (c) Is the cause of stress incontinence of urine.
    (d) May lead to urinary infection.
    (e) Is very uncommon in nulliparous women.

81 The following substances may be secreted by ovarian tumours:
    (a) TSH.
    (b) Serotonin.
    (c) Calmodulin.
    (d) Chorionic gonadotrophin.
    (e) Vasco-active intestinal peptide.

82 The following ovarian tumours are always malignant:
    (a) Myxoma peritonei.
    (b) Endodermal sinus tumour.
    (c) Solid teratoma.
    (d) Granulosa cell tumours.
    (e) Brenner tumours.

77 (a) **True**
   (b) **True** This is called Bonney's test.
   (c) **True** If stress incontinence controllable by Bonney's test is *not* demonstrable during examination, this test should be carried out.
G 244–250
   (d) **False** Cytoscopy has little place in the evaluation of incontinence.
   (e) **True** Surgery should only be considered if incontinence persists for three months after delivery.

78 (a) **False**
   (b) **True**
   (c) **True** **G 62–67**
   (d) **False** It is strikingly uncommon in Negroes, despite high parity.
   (e) **False** Difficulty in defaecation may occur, but not obstruction.

79 (a) **True**
   (b) **False** It is only associated with infertility if there is an underlying cause such as endometriosis or chronic pelvic infection.
   (c) **False** The operation to correct retroversion is a ventrosuspension.
G 68–70
   (d) **False** It is either congenital, acquired following childbirth, or secondary to pelvic adhesions.
   (e) **False** A retroverted uterus only rarely becomes incarcerated in pregnancy and correction with a Hodge pessary is hardly ever indicated.

80 (a) **True**
   (b) **True**
   (c) **False** Although stress incontinence is often associated with cystocele, it is not caused by it. **G 62–64**
   (d) **True** Stasis of urine from any cause may lead to infection.
   (e) **True** It is almost always a consequence of childbirth.

81 (a) **False** Thyroxine is secreted by the *Struma ovarii* of a deimoid cyst.
   (b) **True** Carcinoid syndrome may result.
   (c) **False** This is an intracellular substance. Hypercalcaemia may, however, occur due to parathormone or prostaglandin secretion.
G 142–156
   (d) **True** This is an important 'tumour marker' in choriocarcinoma and endodermal sinus tumour.
   (e) **False**

82 (a) **False** Although spread of benign mucinous cells through the peritoneal cavity is a very serious disorder leading to cachexia, it cannot be regarded as a malignant tumour.
   (b) **True** Potentially this is the most malignant tumour in the human body, but the prognosis has been transformed by chemotherapy.
G 142–156
   (c) **False** If mature tissues predominate, it is benign.
   (d) **False** Only about 30 per cent are malignant. Malignant potential cannot however be reliably predicted from histological appearance.
   (e) **False** These are nearly always benign.

83 Mucin secreting neoplasms of the ovary:
  (a) Are usually malignant.
  (b) Are usually unilocular.
  (c) Can usually be differentiated from simple follicular cysts by ultrasound.
  (d) Are more often bilateral than other ovarian tumours.
  (e) Should always be removed.

84 Carcinoma of the ovary:
  (a) Has a good prognosis if the capsule of the ovary has not been penetrated.
  (b) Is aggravated by oestrogens.
  (c) Is classified as Stage II if it has spread to the pelvic peritoneum.
  (d) Typically spreads across the peritoneal cavity.
  (e) Frequently causes intestinal obstruction.

85 Malignant ovarian disease:
  (a) Is the commonest cause of death from cancer of the reproductive tract in Britain.
  (b) Is usually (FIGO) Stage IV when it is discovered.
  (c) Is staged at operation, unlike cancer of the cervix, which is staged pre-operatively.
  (d) Often presents with amenorrhoea in pre-menopausal patients.
  (e) Is more common in women who have never been pregnant.

86 In the management of cancer of the ovary:
  (a) Chemotherapy is more effective than with other epithelial tumours.
  (b) Progesterone administration may cause a temporary remission.
  (c) Extensive surgery has no place in (FIGO) Stage III carcinoma.
  (d) Dysgerminomas are effectively treated by radiotherapy.
  (e) Only intravenous chemotherapy is effective and oral agents are not useful.

87 Midline incisions are inferior to lower transverse incisions for gynaecological operations in the following respects:
  (a) Exposure is less adequate.
  (b) Incisional hernia is more common.
  (c) Dehiscence of the scar is more likely.
  (d) Wound haematoma is more common.
  (e) The cosmetic result is worse.

83 (a) **False**   Only five to ten per cent are malignant.
    (b) **False**
    (c) **True**   The loculi show up on ultrasound.
    (d) **False**   Only five per cent are bilateral, whilst 50 per cent of serous cystadenocarcinomas are bilateral.   **G 142–155**
    (e) **True**   Unlike simple functional cysts, all neoplasms of the ovary should be removed to exclude malignancy and prevent complications such as torsion or rupture.

84 (a) **True**   Unfortunately ovarian cancer is seldom detected at this early stage. Occasionally, however, such Stage la tumours are discovered by chance at laparotomy for other reasons.
    (b) **False**   It is seldom, if ever, hormone responsive.   **G 153–162**
    (c) **True**
    (d) **True**   This is the most common mode of spread.
    (e) **True**   This is a frequent terminal complication.

85 (a) **True**   It is not, however, the commonest malignancy of the reproductive organs.
    (b) **False**   It is usually Stage III. However, this denotes abdominal spread beyond the pelvic cavity and the prognosis is usually poor.
                                      G 144–156
    (c) **True**
    (d) **False**   Only the rare androgen secreting tumours cause amenorrhoea at an early stage.
    (e) **True**

86 (a) **True**
    (b) **False**   Endometrial carcinoma may have hormone receptors and respond temporarily to progesterone treatment.   **G 160–162**
    (c) **False**   Removal of the bulk of the tumour mass increases the response rate of chemotherapy.
    (d) **True**   They are sensitive to radiotherapy in the same way as seminomas, which they resemble histologically.
    (e) **False**   Although intravenous therapy with cis-platinum is most useful for large tumours, oral alkylating agents such as chlorambucil may be effective in smaller tumours. Oral and intravenous agents may be combined.

87 (a) **False**   It is better and the incision may easily be extended.
    (b) **True**   The rectus sheath should be repaired with a non-absorbable material to lower the incidence of this complication after midline incisions.   **G 267**
    (c) **True**
    (d) **False**   The large exposed areas behind the rectus sheath and on the surface of the rectus abdominus muscles predispose to haematoma formation. The wound is often drained for this reason.
    (e) **True**   The incision cuts across Lange's lines, and therefore leaves a wider scar.

88 The abdominal approach for hysterectomy has the following advantages over vaginal hysterectomy:
   (a) It causes less postoperative pain.
   (b) The ovaries may be removed more easily if an unexpected endometrial cancer is discovered.
   (c) A large uterus is easily removed.
   (d) Prolapse can be repaired more adquately by plicating the uterosacral ligaments.
   (e) Postoperative recovery is more rapid.

89 Anterior colporrhaphy:
   (a) May cause temporary retention of urine.
   (b) Is used in the treatment of stress incontinence.
   (c) Is frequently combined with vaginal hysterectomy.
   (d) Should be avoided in patients with urge incontinence.
   (e) Should not be carried out until childbearing is complete.

90 Dilatation and curettage (D and C):
   (a) Should be carried out in all patients with menorrhagia.
   (b) Should be carried out for all patients with post-menopausal bleeding.
   (c) Should be recommended for all patients with breakthrough bleeding on oral contraception.
   (d) May be helpful in the diagnosis of ectopic pregnancy.
   (e) Is an essential investigation for subfertility.

88 (a) **False** However, if posterior repair is carried out at the time of vaginal hysterectomy, considerable pain will be experienced.

(b) **True** Some surgeons perform a D and C to exclude frank malignancy before performing vaginal hysterectomy. **G 266–267**

(c) **True**

(d) **False** Vaginal hysterectomy with suture of the vault to the cardinal and uterosacral ligaments together with anterior and posterior repair (if required) is the standard operation for prolapse.

(e) **False**

89 (a) **True** Routine postoperative catheterization, preferably with a suprapubic catheter, is often used for this purpose.

(b) **True** However, colposuspension procedures have a higher success rate. **G 265**

(c) **True**

(d) **True** It may make matters worse.

(e) **False** Most surgeons would however recommend delivery by caesarean section after successful anterior colporrhapy.

90 (a) **False** If periods are heavy but still regular and the patient is less than, say, 35 years of age, an endomentrial cancer is so unlikely that D and C is not mandatory.

(b) **True** Even if another cause, such as atrophic vaginitis, is discovered.

(c) **False** It should, however, be carried out if this persists after changing oral contraceptive. **G 263**

(d) **True** Discovery of products of conception almost eliminates an ectopic pregnancy, while the presence of decidua with no trophoblast makes the diagnosis more likely.

(e) **False** Ovulation can now be diagnosed biochemically and a routine endometrial culture for tuberculosis is not essential in Great Britain.

Obstetrics

91 By the time a fetus is mature it is usual for:
   (a) Meconium to have been passed.
   (b) Pulmonary surfactant to have been produced.
   (c) The ductus arteriosus to have closed.
   (d) Hepatic glucuronyl transferase system to be adequate.
   (e) Fetal haemoglobin to be 16–20g/100ml.

92 The denominator (indicator):
   (a) Is the occiput in a flexed cephalic presentation.
   (b) Is the fetal part most closely related to the symphysis pubis.
   (c) Of a face presentation is the submento-bregmatic diameter.
   (d) Of a breech presentation is the sacrum.
   (e) Is used to determine the position.

93 The fetal head:
   (a) Engages by the mento-vertical diameter in face presentations.
   (b) Has a suboccipito-bregmatic diameter of 10.5cm.
   (c) Contains an anterior fontanelle immediately behind the bregma.
   (d) Has one occipital and two frontal bones.
   (e) May be felt abdominally after engagement has taken place.

94 The following terms are appropriate:
   (a) Lie: cephalic.
   (b) Position: flexed.
   (c) Station: at the level of the spines.
   (d) Engagement: two-fifths palpable.
   (e) Presenting part: shoulder.

95 Compared with maternal venous blood, blood in the umbilical vein has:
   (a) Smaller red blood cells.
   (b) A higher haemoglobin concentration.
   (c) A higher haemoglobin saturation.
   (d) A higher oxygen content.
   (e) A higher oxygen partial pressure.

96 Maternal blood flow to the placenta:
   (a) Reaches about 1000ml per minute by the end of pregnancy.
   (b) Is affected by posture.
   (c) Is completely obstructed during the peak of strong contractions.
   (d) Is reduced in pre-eclampsia.
   (e) Is increased by inspiration of 100 per cent oxygen.

91 (a) **False**   If meconium is passed before birth, it is usually a sign of fetal distress.   **OB 15–18**

(b) **True**   This is normally present from the 32nd–34th week of gestation.

(c) **False**   It usually closes some time after birth.

(d) **False**   The inadequacy of this enzyme system is the cause of physiological jaundice.

(e) **True**

92 (a) **True**

(b) **False**   It would be in a direct occipito-anterior position but is not necessarily so. For example, it is the part most closely related to the sacro-iliac joint in an occipito-posterior position. **OB 21–24**

(c) **False**   The chin is the denominator.

(d) **True**

(e) **True**

93 (a) **False**   The mento-vertical diameter is associated with brow presentations and, as it measures 13cm, engagement cannot take place in the term fetus.

(b) **False**   This is the diameter which engages when the head is well flexed and measures 9.5cm.   **OB 21–23**

(c) **False**   The bregma is the point in the middle of the anterior fontanelle.

(d) **True**

(e) **True**   After engagement, two-fifths, one-fifth or none of the head may be felt abdominally.

94 (a) **False**   Cephalic describes presentation.

(b) **False**   Flexion describes the attitude.

(c) **True**   **OB 49–52**

(d) **True**

(e) **True**   The shoulder presents with a transverse lie.

95 (a) **False**   Fetal red cells are larger than those of the adult.

(b) **True**   Eighteen compared with 12 grams per 100ml.

(c) **True**   Eighty compared with 40 per cent.   **OB 17–18**

(d) **True**   Twenty-one compared with 10ml O_2 per 100ml blood.

(e) **False**   The higher haemoglobin concentration and greater oxygen affinity of fetal haemoglobin result in a higher oxygen content despite lower partial pressure.

96 (a) **True**

(b) **True**   Pressure of the uterus on the inferior vena cava in the supine position obstructs venous return from the uterus.

(c) **True**   Venules in the myometrium are completely occluded by surrounding muscle fibres.

(d) **True**   This is an important component of the pathophysiology of pre-eclampsia and may even be the primary event.   **OB 12**

(e) **False**   There is some evidence that it may be decreased, but none that it is increased. Oxygen administration nevertheless is a beneficial temporary measure in fetal distress.

97 By means of real-time ultrasound examination:
    (a) Pregnancy can usually be detected five weeks after the last menstrual period.
    (b) The fetal heart cannot be seen until ten weeks after the last period.
    (c) Placenta praevia can be reliably demonstrated at the 16th week of pregnancy.
    (d) The biparietal diameter can be measured reliably after the 12th week of pregnancy.
    (e) A reliable estimate of gestational age can be made in the third trimester.

98 The fetus:
    (a) Is recognizably human at 12 weeks of gestation.
    (b) Usually weighs over a kilogram at 28 weeks.
    (c) Develops recognizable external genitalia at 14 weeks.
    (d) Can survive hypoxia for longer than an adult.
    (e) Will develop anaemia if the mother is iron-deficient.
    (f) Is most vulnerable to teratogenic agents between ten and 12 weeks.

99 During the development of ovarian follicles:
    (a) The first polar body is extruded before ovulation.
    (b) Meiosis is resumed one week before ovulation.
    (c) The ovum is extruded at the peak of the LH surge.
    (d) Progesterone secretion starts to increase before ovulation.
    (e) Granulosa cells in the corpus luteum are responsible for steroidogenesis.

100 The luteal phase of the menstrual cycle is associated with:
    (a) High progesterone levels.
    (b) High LH levels.
    (c) Low basal body temperature.
    (d) Implantation.
    (e) Rising FSH levels.

101 During normal pregnancy:
    (a) Estradiol is the principal circulating oestrogen.
    (b) The blood pressure falls in the second trimester.
    (c) Blood flow to the liver and kidneys increases by over 25 per cent.
    (d) The pressure of the uterus on the diaphragm reduces the tidal volume and causes dyspnoea.
    (e) The ureters dilate due to obstruction and increased intraluminal pressure.

102 Fibroids in pregnancy:
    (a) Are a recognised cause of obstructed labour.
    (b) Should be removed by myomectomy during pregnancy.
    (c) Should be removed by myomectomy at caesarean section.
    (d) Are likely to regress after the pregnancy.
    (e) May cause acute abdominal pain.

97 (a) **True**   Transvaginal ultrasound detects the gestation sac by 5 weeks, i.e. one week earlier than abdominal ultrasound.

   (b) **False**   It can normally be demonstrated at six to seven weeks by real-time equipment, although ten to 12 weeks are necessary for detection by Doppler.   **OB 54–61**

   (c) **False**   Five to 15 per cent of all pregnancies will have an apparently low placenta at this gestation, as the lower segment has not yet formed to any appreciable degree.

   (d) **True**   It is measurable accurately from 12 weeks' gestation-crown-rump-length is most accurate between eight and 12 weeks.

   (e) **False**   This is the result of the wide range of fetal size for given gestational age at this stage of pregnancy, and the slow rate of growth compared to the inherent range of error of the technique.

98 (a) **True**
   (b) **True**
   (c) **True**   **OB 15–18**
   (d) **True**
   (e) **False**
   (f) **False**   The most critical period is in the early first trimester when most organogenesis occurs.

99 (a) **True**
   (b) **False**   It is resumed 36–48 hours before ovulation.
   (c) **False**   Ovulation occurs 12 hours after the peak and 36 hours after the start of the LH surge.   **OB 1–4**

   (d) **True**
   (e) **True**

100 (a) **True**
    (b) **False**   The LH peak occurs prior to ovulation.
    (c) **False**   The basal temperature rises after ovulation.   **OB 1–4**
    (d) **True**   The blastocyst starts to implant seven days after ovulation.
    (e) **False**   The FSH level rises in the follicular phase.

101 (a) **False**   Estriol is the principal oestrogen.
    (b) **True**
    (c) **False**   Blood flow to the kidneys increases by 30 per cent but splanchnic and hepatic flow is unchanged.   **OB 29–32**
    (d) **False**   Tidal volume is increased due to the effect of progesterone on the respiratory centre.
    (e) **False**   Intraluminal pressure is low; dilatation is due to the smooth muscle relaxant effect of progesterone.

102 (a) **True**   Fibroids situated in the pelvis may obstruct labour, but the growing uterus usually raises them out of the pelvis.
    (b) **False**   There is a high risk of abortion and haemorrhage if myomectomy is attempted in pregnancy.   **OB 64–66**
    (c) **False**   Again, dangerous haemorrhage may occur.
    (d) **True**
    (e) **True**   Degeneration of fibroids is common in pregnancy, causing severe pain.

103 Retroversion of the uterus in pregnancy:
   (a) Is a common cause of recurrent abortion.
   (b) Causes acute retention of urine at the tenth week.
   (c) Should be corrected by the insertion of a Hodge Pessary.
   (d) Usually corrects itself spontaneously after the twelfth week.
   (e) Is often associated with stress incontinence.

104 In ectopic pregnancy:
   (a) Bleeding precedes pain.
   (b) Shoulder tip pain is an important symptom.
   (c) The isthmus of the tube is the commonest site of implantation.
   (d) The incidence is greater in women wearing intra-uterine devices.
   (e) Ultrasonic scan is of no help in diagnosis.

105 Complications of hydatidiform mole include:
   (a) Hyperemesis gravidarum.
   (b) Malignant change.
   (c) Haemorrhage.
   (d) Diabetes insipidus.
   (e) Development of ovarian cysts.

106 First trimester abortion may be due to:
   (a) Inadequate oestrogen production.
   (b) Chromosome abnormality of the fetus.
   (c) Incompetence of the internal cervical os.
   (d) Maternal diabetes.
   (e) Cytotoxic drugs.

107 In eclampsia:
   (a) Large doses of intravenous sedation are given.
   (b) Caesarean section must be carried out, whether the fetus is dead or alive.
   (c) Hypotensive drugs should not be used.
   (d) Ergometrine should be avoided in the third stage of labour.
   (e) Urinary output is increased.

108 In pre-eclamptic toxaemia:
   (a) There is an increase in extra-cellular sodium.
   (b) Proteinurea is the earliest sign.
   (c) Serum uric acid levels tend to decrease.
   (d) The hepatic lesion shows patchy haemorrhage and necrosis.
   (e) There is disturbance of the clotting mechanism.

103 (a) **False**
   (b) **False** It causes retention between the twelfth and sixteenth week.
                                                                            OB 63–64
   (c) **False** This is not generally necessary as the retroversion corrects itself.
   (d) **True**
   (e) **False**

104 (a) **False** Pain usually precedes bleeding.
   (b) **True** Blood tracks up the paracolic gutters to the diaphragm where it causes referred pain.
   (c) **False** The ampulla is the commonest site.   **OB 147–149**
   (d) **True**
   (e) **False** Tubal pregnancy is often identified on transvaginal ultrasonic scan, and the scan is also helpful in excluding an intra-uterine pregnancy when the beta HCG is positive.

105 (a) **True** This is thought to be due to the excessive production of chorionic gonadotrophin.   **OB 68–70**
   (b) **True** Two to ten per cent progress to choriocarcinoma, the incidence varying in different parts of the world.
   (c) **True** Expulsion of the mole or surgical evacuation may be associated with haemorrhage.
   (d) **False**
   (e) **True** Theca lutein cysts of the ovary may develop due to stimulation by chorionic gonadotrophin.

106 (a) **False** This theory has been discredited.
   (b) **True** Some 60 per cent of abortion material has been found to be chromosomally abnormal.   **OB 142–146**
   (c) **False** Cervical imcompetence causes mid-trimester abortion.
   (d) **True** Poorly controlled diabetes may cause abortion.
   (e) **True**

107 (a) **True**
   (b) **False** If the fetus is dead or the cervix very favourable, induction of labour may be attempted.
   (c) **False** Hypotensives are used to reduce the risk of cerebral haemorrhage.   **OB 91–93**
   (d) **True** The vasoconstrictor effect raises the blood pressure; syntocinon is preferable.
   (e) **False** There is oliguria (which may progress to renal failure).

108 (a) **True** There is retention of both water and sodium.
   (b) **False** Weight gain, oedema and hypertension usually precede proteinurea.   **OB 87–90**
   (c) **False** Levels increase as a result of an alteration in renal tubular function.
   (d) **True**
   (e) **True** There is a fall in platelets, and an increased level of fibrin degradation products.

109 There is an increased risk of developing pre-eclampsia with:
  (a) Increasing maternal age.
  (b) High parity.
  (c) Hydatidiform mole.
  (d) Maternal cardiac disease.
  (e) Diabetes.

110 Coagulation failure is an important complication of:
  (a) Placenta praevia.
  (b) Abruptio placentae.
  (c) Amniotic fluid embolus.
  (d) Gram-negative septicaemia.
  (e) Uterine rupture.

111 The following may cause intra-uterine death of the fetus:
  (a) Diabetes mellitus.
  (b) Respiratory distress syndrome (RDS).
  (c) Hydrops fetalis.
  (d) A sudden emotional shock to the mother.
  (e) Syphilis.

112 When intra-uterine death of the fetus occurs in the third trimester:
  (a) Caesarean section should be carried out to deliver the fetus.
  (b) There is a tendency to thrombo-embolism.
  (c) There is a danger of anaerobic infection.
  (d) Lactation will not occur after delivery.
  (e) The birth of the baby must be registered.

113 Hydramnios is associated with the following:
  (a) Chorio-angioma of the placenta.
  (b) Maternal diabetes.
  (c) Hydatidiform mole.
  (d) Hydrops fetalis.
  (e) Intra-uterine growth retardation of the fetus.

114 Oligohydramnios is associated with the following fetal conditions:
  (a) Tracheo-oesophageal fistula.
  (b) Talipes.
  (c) Potter's syndrome.
  (d) Intra-uterine growth retardation.
  (e) Anencephaly.

115 The incidence of multiple pregnancy is increased:
  (a) In people of Negro race.
  (b) In women treated with bromocriptine for infertility.
  (c) In women treated by *in vitro* fertilization.
  (d) With advancing maternal age.
  (e) First pregnancies.

109 (a) **True**
   (b) **False** It is most common in primigravidae.
   (c) **True**   **OB 89**
   (d) **False**
   (e) **True**

110 (a) **False** There is straightforward haemorrhage in this condition.
   (b) **True**   Disseminated intravascular coagulation is thought to occur possibly as a result of thromboplastin release from the placental site.   **OB 266–268**
   (c) **True**   There is widespread disseminated intravascular coagulation.
   (d) **True**   Endotoxins stimulate the clotting mechanism along with many other systems such as complement and kinins. This is particularly likely to occur in pregnancy.
   (e) **False**

111 (a) **True**   Poorly controlled diabetes may lead to sudden fetal death.
   (b) **False** This is a cause of neonatal death.   **OB 133–136**
   (c) **True**
   (d) **False** This only occurs in fiction!
   (e) **True**

112 (a) **False** Vaginal delivery is much to be preferred.
   (b) **False** Hypofibrinogenaemia may occur resulting in failure of blood coagulation.   **OB 133–136**
   (c) **True**   Once the membranes have ruptured there is an ideal culture medium for anaerobic organisms.
   (d) **False** Suppression of lactation should be considered.
   (e) **True**   It must be registered as a stillbirth.

113 (a) **True**
   (b) **True**
   (c) **False** The uterus is filled with molar tissue.   **OB 84–85**
   (d) **True**
   (e) **False** It is often associated with oligohydramnios.

114 (a) **False** This causes hydramnios due to failure of swallowing.
   (b) **True**   Limb deformations occur because of local pressure.
   (c) **True**   Renal agenesis results in lack of liquor.   **OB 85–86**
   (d) **True**
   (e) **False** Often associated with hydramnios due to inability of fetus to swallow.

115 (a) **True**
   (b) **False** Bromocriptine does not induce multiple ovulation.
   (c) **True**   The replacement of several embryos leads to a greater risk of multiple pregnancy.   **OB 136–137**
   (d) **True**
   (e) **False** It is commonest in multigravid women.

116 In twin delivery:
  (a) The first twin is at greater risk than the second.
  (b) Labour usually occurs before term.
  (c) Epidural analgesia is best avoided.
  (d) There is an increased risk of post-partum haemorrhage.
  (e) The commonest presentation is one cephalic, one breech.

117 Ante-partum haemorrhage:
  (a) Is defined as 'bleeding from the genital tract in pregnancy'.
  (b) May be complicated by hypofibrinogenaemia.
  (c) Requires assessment by vaginal examination.
  (d) May be caused by cervical carcinoma.
  (e) Is always painless.

118 To prevent rhesus disease iso-immunization anti-D should be given to rhesus negative women:
  (a) Within 72 hours of delivery of a rhesus positive child.
  (b) Who are known to have rhesus antibodies, within 72 hours of delivery.
  (c) Following a termination of pregnancy, even when the father is known to be heterozygous.
  (d) When an external cephalic version has been performed.
  (e) When an ultrasonic scan has been performed.

119 In rhesus iso-immunization the following tests may be helpful:
  (a) Rhesus antibody titre in liquor.
  (b) Liquor bilirubin level.
  (c) Maternal serum bilirubin.
  (d) Direct Coombs' test on cord blood.
  (e) Rhesus genotype of husband.

120 Maternal mortality:
  (a) Now stands at a rate of 0.1 per thousand total births.
  (b) Does not include deaths from therapeutic abortion.
  (c) Must be reported to the Coroner.
  (d) Is subjected to a Confidential Enquiry.
  (e) Is most often caused by sepsis.

121 Post-partum haemorrhage:
  (a) Is defined as a blood loss of one litre.
  (b) Is less likely if oxytocics are administered routinely in the third stage of labour.
  (c) Is 'primary' if it occurs within the first 12 hours.
  (d) Is common after both placenta praevia and abruptio placentae.
  (e) May require manual removal of the placenta.

116 (a) **False** Fetal mortality and morbidity is greater in the second twin.
  (b) **True** Over-distension of the uterus leads to pre-term labour.
OB 139–141
  (c) **False** Epidural analgesia is ideal, in preparation for any second-stage difficulties.
  (d) **True**
  (e) **False** The commonest presentation is cephalic-cephalic (45 per cent).

117 (a) **False** It is bleeding from the genital tract after fetal viability (c. 24 weeks).
  (b) **True** This occurs in placental abruption, due to release of thromboplastins from the placenta.
  (c) **False** Vaginal examination is dangerous until placenta praevia has been ruled out. **OB 74–83**
  (d) **True** This is an "incidental" cause of A.P.H.
  (e) **False** Placental abruption is usually painful, whilst bleeding from placenta praevia is painless.

118 (a) **True**
  (b) **False** Giving anti-D once there are rhesus antibodies is a useless exercise.
  (c) **True** A heterozygous father has a 50 per cent chance of producing a rhesus positive offspring. **OB 322**
  (d) **True** The trauma of version may produce feto-maternal haemorrhage.
  (e) **False** There is insufficient trauma to cause feto-maternal haemorrhage.

119 (a) **False** Rhesus antibody titre in *maternal blood* is done periodically to assess the likelihood of the fetus being affected.
  (b) **True** This is usually done spectro-photometrically on liquor obtained at an amniocentesis. **OB 320–321**
  (c) **False** The maternal bilirubin is not altered.
  (d) **True** This test confirms whether the baby is affected.
  (e) **True** If the husband is heterozygous, there is a 50 per cent chance that the offspring will not be affected.

120 (a) **True**
  (b) **False** Deaths from abortion, both spontaneous and therapeutic are included. **OB 340–344**
  (c) **False** The same regulations relate to reporting to the Coroner as with any kind of death.
  (d) **True**
  (e) **False** Hypertension and pulmonary embolus are the biggest causes of death.

121 (a) **False** 500 to 600 ml. is a more usual figure.
  (b) **True** This has been confirmed by several randomised trials.
  (c) **False** Secondary post-partum haemorrhage occurs after 24 hours.
  (d) **True** In placenta praevia, large placental vessels are surrounded by relatively thin and poorly contractile lower uterine segment which is unable to provide effective occlusive power. In abruptio placenta, i) the bruised 'couvelaire' uterus tends to remain hypotonic, and ii) consumptive coagulopathy is often present.
OB 228–233
  (e) **True**

122 The following are always indications for caesarean section:
   (a) Hydrocephalus.
   (b) Grade 4 placenta praevia.
   (c) Abruptio placentae.
   (d) Untreated Stage Ib cancer of the cervix.
   (e) Active primary genital herpes.

123 During vaginal breech delivery:
   (a) Episiotomy should be carried out immediately before delivery of the head.
   (b) There is a risk that the 'after coming' head may be retained by a rim of cervix.
   (c) Traction on the anterior groin should be used if the breech does not enter the pelvis in the second stage.
   (d) Løvset's maneouvre should always be carried out.
   (e) Pre-existing hypoxia is no more dangerous than it would be with vertex delivery.

124 Obstructed labour:
   (a) Always develops before full dilatation of the cervix.
   (b) Can usually be predicted before the onset of labour.
   (c) Is more common in developed countries.
   (d) Is inevitable in a term fetus with persistent mento-posterior position.
   (e) Can often be overcome by means of craniotomy if the fetus is dead.

125 The following are correct associations:
   (a) Anencephaly – face presentation.
   (b) Advancing maternal age – Turner's syndrome.
   (c) Hydatidiform mole – pre-eclampsia.
   (d) Diabetes mellitus – neonatal hyperglycaemia.
   (e) Precipitate labour – post-partum haemorrhage.

126 Fetal tachycardia:
   (a) May be the result of previous maternal thyrotoxicosis.
   (b) Usually has a good prognosis if base-line variability is retained.
   (c) Is more common after prolonged rupture of the membranes.
   (d) Seldom exceeds 200 beats per minute.
   (e) May occur in severe rhesus disease.

122 (a) **False**   The hydrocephalus can usually be decompressed transcervically or by ultrasound directed transcutaneous methods.

  (b) **True**   This is the safest method of delivery, even if the fetus is dead.
OB 289

  (c) **False**   The baby is often dead in these cases and vaginal delivery is preferable if labour progresses rapidly.

  (d) **True**   Delivery disseminates cancer cells.

  (e) **True**   Primary genital herpes may infect the infant during birth. This causes encephalitis and has a high mortality.

123 (a) **False**   It should be carried out when the buttock distends the perineum.

  (b) **True**   This is particularly likely with a premature or footling breech.

  (c) **False**   If the breech remains high, caesarean section is indicated. This suggests pelvic disproportion and the head is likely to be obstructed or damaged if the breech is delivered vaginally.
OB 195–198

  (d) **False**   This is carried out for nuchal displacement of the arms.

  (e) **False**   A degree of asphyxia is inevitable in vaginal breech delivery because the cord is obstructed once the chest enters the pelvis. This can only be tolerated if the fetus is well oxygenated prior to delivery.

124 (a) **False**   In most cases of obstructed labour, cervical dilatation is slow and full dilatation may never occur. In others, the patient proceeds to full dilatation without dealy, and is then unable to deliver the fetus.

  (b) **False**   In some cases, for example those with a bony deformity of the pelvis, this can be predicted. In most cases, however, it is impossible to predict the outcome of labour with any accuracy.
OB 209–211

  (c) **False**   The mean pelvic size is smaller in non-developed countries.

  (d) **True**   The mento-posterior position usually results in a rotation through three-eighths of a circle which permits delivery in the mento-anterior position. If this fails to occur, there is no mechanism for delivery and manual rotation, Kielland's forceps or caesarean section is required.

  (e) **True**   Craniotomy will be effective if the fetus is presenting by the vertex; more complex destructive operations or Caesarean section are required for an impacted, dead transverse lie.

125 (a) **True**

  (b) **False**   Unlike autosomal trisomies, Turner's syndrome becomes *less* common with advancing age.

  (c) **True**

  (d) **False**   Hypoglycaemia is a problem because of fetal hyperinsulinaemia.

  (e) **True**

126 (a) **True**   Long-acting thyroid stimulating antibodies may still be present.

  (b) **True**

  (c) **True**   This is due to the resulting amnionitis and pyrexia.

  (d) **True**   Only fetal arrythmia will exceed this rate.   **OB 216–220**

  (e) **True**   A fast flat trace occurs in acute blood loss or chronic anaemia due to immune haemolytic disease.

127 Spontaneous pre-term labour:
    (a) Multiple pregnancy is the commonest cause.
    (b) Is defined as labour before the 34th week.
    (c) Does not tend to recur in subsequent pregnancies.
    (d) Is the commonest cause of perinatal mortality.
    (e) Is common in pre-eclampsia.

128 Symptoms and signs of the onset of labour include:
    (a) Braxton Hicks contractions.
    (b) Absent fetal movement.
    (c) Shortening of the cervix.
    (d) Dilatation of the cervix.
    (e) Spinnbarkeit.

129 Uterine contractions in labour:
    (a) Start at the cornu.
    (b) Involve uterine muscle retraction.
    (c) Are painful due to ischaemia.
    (d) Are efficient at 5mm. Hg.
    (e) Are consciously controllable.

130 Fetal monitoring in labour:
    (a) Shows the normal heart rate to be 120–160 beats/min.
    (b) May involve checking the fetal pH.
    (c) Is mandatory.
    (d) Looks for beat to beat variations.
    (e) Measures uterine activity and heart rate.

131 Active management of the third stage:
    (a) Involves the Matthews Duncan method.
    (b) May involve intra-venous syntocinon.
    (c) Increases the risk of needing a manual removal.
    (d) Increases the chance of post-partum haemorrhage.
    (e) Begins with delivery of the fetal trunk.

132 The second stage of labour:
    (a) Causes a transient bradycardia with contractions which are of little significance.
    (b) Is less painful than the first.
    (c) Ends with placental separation.
    (d) Starts with pushing.
    (e) Is shorter in multipara.

133 The third stage of labour:
    (a) Starts early in the second stage.
    (b) Ends with placental separation.
    (c) Ends uterine activity.
    (d) Generally involves > 200mls. blood loss.
    (e) Involves retraction of uterine muscle.

127 (a) **False**   Unexplained is by far the most common cause.
   (b) **False**   It is defined as labour before the 37th week. However, no attempt is made to stop labour after the 34th or 35th week.
                                                    OB 212–214
   (c) **False**   A previous history of premature delivery is a strong risk factor for another premature delivery.
   (d) **True**
   (e) **False**   However, early labour is often induced for this reason.

128 (a) **False**   These may be felt throughout pregnancy as painless, irregular contractions.
   (b) **False**   Absence of fetal movements should always be regarded with suspicion.   **OB 151–154**
   (c) **True**
   (d) **True**
   (e) **False**   This is a change in the cervical mucus seen at ovulation.

129 (a) **True**
   (b) **True**
   (c) **True**   **OB 152–155**
   (d) **False**   Contractions are not palpable when less than 20mm/Hg., and efficient contractions reach a pressure of 50mm/Hg.
   (e) **False**

130 (a) **True**
   (b) **True**
   (c) **False**   Low risk normal mothers need intermittent ausculation only.
                                                    OB 164–166
   (d) **True**   Lack of beat-to-beat variation may indicate fetal distress.
   (e) **True**   Both uterine activity and fetal heart rate may be measured either externally or internally.

131 (a) **False**   This is a description of the passive delivery of the placenta.
   (b) **True**
   (c) **True**   **OB 170–172**
   (d) **False**   The use of oxytocics and active management reduces the risk of PPH.
   (e) **False**   It begins with an injection of an oxytocic agent with the delivery of the anterior shoulder.

132 (a) **True**   There are often decelerations due to head compression.
   (b) **True**
   (c) **False**   **OB 155–156**
   (e) **False**   Full dilatation of the cervix marks the onset of the second stage, but the urge to push may not be felt until the head is on the pelvic floor.
   (e) **True**

133 (a) **False**   It starts when the fetus has been delivered.   **OB 156–157**
   (c) **False**   Uterine retraction continues into the puerperium.
   (d) **False**   Mean blood loss is less than 200mls.
   (e) **True**

134 The following predispose to primary post-partum haemorrhage:
   (a) Administration of prolonged or deep anaesthesia to the mother.
   (b) Twin pregnancy.
   (c) Oligohydramnios.
   (d) Prolonged labour caused by mechanical difficulty.
   (e) Hyperemesis gravidarum.

135 Concerning third stage traumatic lesions:
   (a) Repair of a third degree perineal tear should not be attempted using only local anaesthesia.
   (b) A second degree tear involves the perineal body and includes the anal sphincter.
   (c) An extensive tear of the vagina can occur without a tear in the perineum.
   (d) The symptoms of fistulae resulting from pressure necrosis during prolonged labour appear immediately after delivery.
   (e) Fistuale resulting from direct trauma (e.g. during Caesarean section or craniotomy) should not be repaired for two to three months.

136 The following are contra-indications to intravenous beta adrenergic stimulant therapy in obstetric practice:
   (a) Pre-term labour.
   (b) Fetal distress in labour.
   (c) Previous caesarean section.
   (d) Asthma.
   (e) Insulin dependent diabetes.

137 The following are absolute contra-indications to epidural analgesia:
   (a) Hypertrophic obstructive cardiomyopathy.
   (b) Pilonidal sinus.
   (c) Abruptio placentae.
   (d) Pre-term labour.
   (e) Twins.

134 (a) **True**
    (b) **True**   Overdistension of the uterus predisposes to failure of retraction.
    (c) **False**
    (d) **True**   Incoordinate uterine action occurs after prolonged labour.
                                        OB 228–229
    (e) **False**

135 (a) **True**
    (b) **False**   Laceration of the anal sphincter places the tear into the category of the third degree.
    (c) **True**   **OB 226–227**
    (d) **False**   The symptoms frequently do not appear for 10 days.
    (e) **False**

136 (a) **False**   This is the primary indication for this therapy.
    (b) **False**   Uterine contractions obstruct placental blood flow and it is the asphyxia, in an already compromised fetus, that causes distress. Abolition of contractions by beta stimulant therapy is therefore beneficial while arranging measures for delivery.
                                        OB 212–214
    (c) **False**
    (d) **False**   This is an indication for beta andrenergic stimulant therapy. Cardiac disease, especially aortic and mitral stenosis, are contra-indications.
    (e) **True**   The insulin requirement increases by about five times on this treatment and the disease becomes difficult to control. This effect is further aggravated if steroids are given to hasten fetal lung maturity.

137 (a) **True**   In this condition, any reduction in end diastolic volume narrows the ventricular outflow tract and aggravates failure. The reduced left ventricular pressures will increase the shunt in Eisenmenger's syndrome and this is therefore also an absolute contra-indication. Other forms of heart disease may benefit from epidural analgesia because the increased cardiac output caused by pain and fright is diminished.   **OB 173–174**
    (b) **True**   Any local sepsis will predispose to an epidural abscess.
    (c) **True**   (i) Shock is likely to be aggravated by abolishing protective vasoconstriction. (ii) Bleeding may occur into the epidural space as a result of consumptive coagulopathy.
    (d) **False**   By avoiding the use of drugs which inhibit respiration, this technique may be especially suited for premature labour.
    (e) **False**   Epidural analgesia is suitable for twin delivery and will allow a rapid delivery to be effected if fetal distress, cord prolapse or other complications occur after delivery of the first twin.

138 Syntocinon augmentation of labour:
  (a) Is more often required in multiparous patients.
  (b) Aggravates fetal distress.
  (c) May cause a prolonged hypertonic uterine contraction.
  (d) May have to be reduced as labour progresses.
  (e) May cause or aggravate neonatal jaundice.

139 Fetal distress during the first stage of labour:
  (a) Always causes Type II dips. (late decelerations)
  (b) Can be diagnosed with a high degree of confidence if meconium is present.
  (c) Is associated with an accumulation of lactic acid in the fetus.
  (d) Should be treated with an infusion of bicarbonate.
  (e) Can be helped by oxygen and glucose in the short term, while making preparations for caesarean section.

140 The following predispose to fetal distress in labour:
  (a) The supine position.
  (b) Pre-eclampsia.
  (c) Renal disease.
  (d) Lupus erythematosus.
  (e) Pethidine administration.

141 Prior to engagement of the fetal head:
  (a) The vertex may be visible at the vulva.
  (b) A trial of forceps may be carried out provided that the vertex has passed the plane of the pelvic inlet.
  (c) Three-fifths or more of the head are palpable abdominally.
  (d) Induction of labour should not be carried out.
  (e) Spontaneous labour is unlikely to start.

138 (a) **False** Hypotonic inertia in the absence of disproportion is commoner in primiparous patients.

(b) **True** Uterine contractions always obstruct placental blood flow. They become stronger with syntocinon and the recovery phase between contractions is shortened.

(c) **True** This causes fetal distress, and may cause uterine rupture.
OB 180–181

(d) **True** Labour is a self-perpetuating process and the dose may have to be reduced if contractions occur too frequently as this will cause fetal asphyxia.

(e) **True** This may be due in part to the anti-diuretic effect of oxytocin causing red cells to swell and become less distensible. Such cells are more rapidly removed from the circulation.

139 (a) **False** It usually causes Type II dips. Unfortunately, severe fetal distress can occur with a normal cardiotocograph trace. This accounts for about ten per cent of cases of fetal distress. Similarly, only one half to two-thirds of fetuses with Type II dips are hypoxic at birth. **OB 216–221**

(b) **False** Most often, the passage of meconium is not associated with fetal distress. Nevertheless, meconium is a warning sign which increases the likelihood of fetal distress.

(c) **True** Fetal distress is usually caused by hypoxia. This causes anaerobic metabolism and lactate accumulation.

(d) **False** Although the fetus is acidotic, bicarbonate is not helpful as it does not cross the placenta well. It also shifts the mother's oxygen dissociation curve to the left, which may further aggravate fetal hypoxia.

(e) **False** Oxygen is of benefit but glucose compounds lactate accumulation and hastens fetal death.

140 (a) **True** Pressure on the inferior vena cava diminishes venous return from the placenta. **OB 216–221**

(b) **True** ⎫ Narrowing of the spiral arteries together with vasospasm
(c) **True** ⎭ diminish placental blood flow.

(d) **True** Patients with the 'lupus anti-coagulant' develop micro-thrombi in the placental circulation.

(e) **False** This predisposes to poor respiratory effort after delivery.

141 (a) **True** This is unusual but possible, especially when (i) the head is highly moulded, and (ii) the pelvis is very shallow – this is seen particularly in the negro pelvis. **OB 205–209**

(b) **False** This is still a high forceps and should not be carried out.

(c) **True**

(d) **False**

(e) **False** In 60 per cent of multiparous and 40 per cent of primiparous patients the head does not engage prior to labour.

142 Prolapse of the umbilical cord:
   (a) May occur while the membranes are still intact.
   (b) Is a risk of induction of labour with prostaglandin pessaries.
   (c) Has an incidence of one per cent of labours.
   (d) Is more common in singleton than in twin deliveries.
   (e) Causes severe respiratory acidosis in the fetus.

143 The occipito-posterior position:
   (a) Is an example of a malpresentation.
   (b) Usually turns to deliver as the occipito-anterior position.
   (c) May proceed to deep transverse arrest.
   (d) Is associated with a prolonged first stage.
   (e) Is associated with a prolonged second stage.

144 Hyperthyroidism in pregnancy:
   (a) Should be treated surgically rather than with carbimazole.
   (b) May lead to neonatal hyperthyroidism even though the mother's disease is treated.
   (c) Should not be treated with anti-thyroid drugs.
   (d) Can be diagnosed by total T4 measurement.
   (e) Is always associated with increased long acting thyroid stimulator.

145 Anaemia in pregnancy:
   (a) Is defined as haemoglobin of 10.0G or less.
   (b) May be caused by haemodilution of pregnancy.
   (c) May be caused by hookworm infestation.
   (d) When megaloblastic, is usually due to B12 deficiency.
   (e) Is relatively common in multiple pregnancy.

146 In iron deficiency anaemia in pregnancy:
   (a) Mean corpuscular haemoglobin content and mean corpuscular concentration are both low.
   (b) Mean corpuscular volume (MCV) is raised.
   (c) Blood transfusion is indicated if haemoglobin levels fall to below 9.0G.
   (d) There is usually a chronic blood loss causing the anaemia.
   (e) There is an increased risk of pre-eclampsia.

142 (a) **False** A cord below the presenting part but in an intact bag of membranes is a cord presentation.
  (b) **False** It is a risk of surgical induction with a high presenting part or in the presence of hydramnios. **OB 214–215**
  (c) **False** 0.3 per cent would be a more accurate figure.
  (d) **False** It is very common with the second twin, especially if the membranes rupture (or are ruptured) before contractions resume and the presenting part descends.
  (e) **True** This is the initial effect of rapidly accumulating carbon dioxide. Later the hypoxia will lead to a super-imposed metabolic acidosis.

143 (a) **False** It is a malposition. Breech and face are malpresentations.
  (b) **True** This happens in 90 per cent of cases.
  (c) **True** This happens when anterior rotation of the occiput is arrested in the transverse position. **OB 182–186**
  (d) **True** Contractions are often less effective. The head tends to be deflexed and engage by the sub-occipito frontal (10cm) diameter.
  (e) **True** Rotation takes place in the late first and second stages.

144 (a) **True** Carbimazole will usually control the disease adequately.
  (b) **True** Long acting thyroid is a gamma globulin which may cross the placenta and give rise to fetal hyperthyroidism.
  (c) **False** Although carbimazole and propylthiouracil cross the placenta, they do not cause fetal hypothroidism if cautiously administered. **OB 121**
  (d) **False** Total thyroxine is raised in pregnancy and free thyroxine levels or a suppressed TRH test are necessary for biochemical diagnosis.
  (e) **False** Long acting thyroid stimulator is only rarely present.

145 (a) **False** It is defined as haemoglobin level of less than 11.0G. The anaemia is not necessarily pathological but may be physiological due to dilution. **OB 102–104**
  (b) **True** The plasma volume may increase by 30 per cent or more, resulting in a dilutional anaemia, despite an increase in red cell mass.
  (c) **True**
  (d) **False** B12 deficiency is very rare in pregnancy and megaloblastic anaemia is usually due to folic acid deficiency.
  (e) **True** This is a result of dilution, and increased iron and folate requirements.

146 (a) **True** This is a differentiating feature from beta-thalassaemia, where the MCH is low but the MCHC is normal.
  (b) **False** The MCV is low, with hypochromasia. **OB 103–104**
  (c) **False** Blood transfusion is only indicated if the patient is near term, and so there is insufficient time to raise the heamoglobin with iron therapy.
  (d) **False** Inadequate dietary iron is the usual cause.
  (e) **False** There is no relationship between anaemia and pre-eclampsia.

147 In sickle-cell disorders:
(a) There is failure of formation of the β chain of haemoglobin.
(b) The haemoglobin level rarely falls below 9.0G.
(c) There is a high incidence in Negroes and Asians.
(d) Iron deficiency is usual
(e) Crisis is unlikely to occur with the trait.

148 Diabetes mellitus in pregnancy is associated with the following:
(a) Increased incidence of congenital defects.
(b) Increased insulin requirements.
(c) Increased risk of placental abruption.
(d) High incidence of vaginal Trichomonas infection.
(e) Fetal macrosomia.

149 In acute pyelonephritis in pregnancy:
(a) The left kidney is affected more often than the right.
(b) The temperature rarely exceeds 39°C.
(c) Antibiotics should be started before bacteriological results are available.
(d) The incidence of fetal growth retardation and pre-term labour is increased.
(e) Intravenous pyelography should be carried out promptly.

150 In cardiac disease in pregnancy:
(a) Congenital heart disease is the commonest cause.
(b) Cardiac failure should not be treated with digoxin.
(c) Delivery should be by planned caesarean section.
(d) Cardiac surgery is absolutely contra-indicated.
(e) Ergometrine should be avoided in the third stage.

151 Congenital malformations can be attributed to maternal infection with:
(a) Poliomyelitis.
(b) Toxoplasmosis.
(c) Measles.
(d) Cytomegalovirus.
(e) Chicken pox.

147 (a) **False**   It is thalassaemia that is caused by defective β chain formation:
In sickle-cell haemoglobin there is alteration in the amino acid
structure of the chain.

   (b) **False**   Severe anaemia may occur in sickle cell disease.

OB 104–106

   (c) **False**   There is a high incidence in Negroes, but not in Asians.

   (d) **False**   Iron stores are usually adequate.

   (e) **True**   The concentration of HbS is usually too low for sickling to occur.

148 (a) **True**

   (b) **True**

   (c) **False**   **OB 110–112**

   (d) **False**   It is vaginal Candida infection which is associated with diabetes.

   (e) **True**

149 (a) **False**   The right kidney is affected more often than the left.

   (b) **False**   Fevers of 39.5°C and above are common, and often associated
with rigors.   **OB 97–106**

   (c) **True**

   (d) **True**

   (e) **False**   It is only indicated for recurrent attacks of unilateral pyelonephritis, and even then is usually deferred until six weeks post-
partum.

150 (a) **False**   Rheumatic heart disease remains the commonest cause.

   (b) **False**   Digoxin is perfectly safe in pregnancy, although its efficiency in
some forms of cardiac disease is minimal (e.g. mitral stenosis
unless atrial fibrillation is also present).   **OB 106–109**

   (c) **False**   Caesarean section is only advised for obstetric reasons.

   (d) **False**   Cardio-pulmonary bypass and open-heart surgery carries a
considerable risk of fetal loss, but closed heart surgery may be
carried out with reasonable safety.

   (e) **True**   Ergometrine, by causing an increase in blood pressure and
venous return, may precipitate cardiac failure.

151 (a) **False**

   (b) **True**   Blindness, hydrocephaly and mental deficiency have all been
reported.   **OB 113–115**

   (c) **False**

   (d) **True**   Although the majority of babies are not affected, mental retardation and deafness may occur.

   (e) **False**   Congenital infection may however occur if the mother has
chicken-pox shortly before delivery.

152 The following drugs are known to be teratogenic:
  (a) Phenobarbitone.
  (b) Valium.
  (c) Alpha methyldopa.
  (d) Erythromycin.
  (e) Thiazide diuretics.

153 During pregnancy, the following conditions are usually exacerbated:
  (a) Peptic ulcer.
  (b) Multiple sclerosis.
  (c) Meralgia parasthetica.
  (d) Asthma.
  (e) Psoriasis.

154 Asymptomatic bacteruria in early pregnancy:
  (a) Is found in at least ten per cent of women at booking.
  (b) Is only regarded as significant when the bacterial count is more than 10^6 organisms per ml.
  (c) Leads in later pregnancy to pyelonephritis in 30 per cent of cases.
  (d) Should not be treated until the second trimester.
  (e) Is usually caused by *Strep. faecalis.*

155 The following predispose to deep venous thrombosis:
  (a) Caesarean section.
  (b) Antenatal bed rest.
  (c) Breast feeding.
  (d) Varicose veins.
  (e) Pelvic infection.

156 After delivery:
  (a) A vulvovaginal haematoma should not be incised for fear of causing an abscess.
  (b) Third degree tear usually leads to rectal incontinence despite immediate suture.
  (c) Bimanual compression is useful to expel a retained placenta.
  (d) A much more concentrated oxytocin infusion may be administered than would ever be used in labour.
  (e) Only one 0.5mg ampoule of ergometrine may be administered within the first hour.

152 (a) **False**   Phenytoin, which is often given with phenobarbitone for epilepsy, is occasionally associated with chondrodysplasia punctata but this is not an indication to stop the drug. Folate should be given with phenytoin.   **OB 46–49**

   (b) **False**   Valium may however depress respiration in the neonate.

   (c) **False**   This drug and beta blockers are the most widely used for hypertension in pregnancy.

   (d) **False**   Erythromycin, penicillin and cephalosporins are safe in pregnancy. (Sulphonamides may aggravate neontal jaundice, tetracylines damage teeth and bones, aminoglycosides occasionally damage the VIIIth nerve and trimethoprim antagonizes folate and therefore provides a theoretical teratogenic risk).

   (e) **False**   They may, however, aggravate neonatal thrombocytopenia.

153 (a) **False**

   (b) **False**   Relapse may occur after delivery.

   (c) **True**   This condition is caused by entrapment of the lateral cutaneous nerve of the thigh.   **OB 119–122**

   (d) **False**   It often improves, possibly due to increased corticosteroid production.

   (e) **False**

154 (a) **False**   The incidence is three to six per cent.

   (b) **False** 10^5 organisms is usually significant and warrants treatment or further counts.   **OB 97–98**

   (c) **True**

   (d) **False**   It should be treated as soon as possible as this reduces the incidence of pyelonephritis.

   (e) **False**   *Escherichia Coli* is the infective organism in 80 per cent of cases.

155 (a) **True**   Abdonimal delivery considerably increases the risk of thromboembolism.   **OB 268–270**

   (b) **True**

   (c) **False**   Suppression of lactation with oestrogen predisposes to thrombosis.

   (d) **False**   Varicose veins increase the risk of *superficial* thrombophlebitis.

   (e) **True**

156 (a) **False**   If tense, painful or enlarging, it is best decompressed and the bleeding vessel ligated or oversown.

   (b) **False**   The prognosis is excellent with adequate repair.

   (c) **False**   A retained placenta should be removed manually. Bimanual compression is useful for atonic post-partum haemorrhage.   **OB 226–234**

   (d) **True**   In the treatment of atonic post-partum haemorrhage, doses such as 50 units in 500ml may be given at 30–60 drops per minute without the danger of uterine rupture that exists before delivery.

   (e) **False**   A maximum of two 0.5mg dosages may be given in the case of severe atonic post-partum haemorrhage.

157 The following organisms are recognised causes of puerperal pelvic sepsis:
    (a) *Escherichia coli.*
    (b) Haemolytic streptoccocus (Group A).
    (c) *Haemophilus influenzae.*
    (d) *Clostridium welchii.*
    (e) *Staphylococcus aureus.*

158 Puerperal sepsis due to *Haemolytic streptococcus* (Group A):
    (a) May cause rigors;
    (b) Is the commonest cause of maternal mortality.
    (c) Is likely to be caused by endogenous infection.
    (d) Haemoglobinuria is usual.
    (e) Is treated with tetracycline.

159 Breast feeding has the following advantages over bottle feeding:
    (a) Human milk contains more protein.
    (b) Human milk contains more carbohydrate.
    (c) There is a lower incidence of cot death in breast fed infants.
    (d) There is a lower incidence of atopic conditions.
    (e) It needs to be given less frequently.

160 Engorgement of the breasts in a lactating mother is treated by:
    (a) Stopping feeding for 24 hours.
    (b) Giving diuretics.
    (c) Manual or mechanical expression.
    (d) Discarding brassieres.
    (e) Analgesics.

161 In puerperal breast abscess:
    (a) Streptococci are the most common infecting organism.
    (b) Suppression of lactation is advisable.
    (c) Surgical drainage is rarely necessary.
    (d) The whole breast is affected.
    (e) Antibiotics should always be given.

162 Small for dates babies are particularly liable to develop:
    (a) Hypoglycaemia.
    (b) Hypothermia.
    (c) Respiratory distress syndrome (RDS).
    (d) Anaemia.
    (e) Pneumonia.

163 Cephalhaematoma:
    (a) Is caused by oedema of the subcutaneous layers of the scalp.
    (b) Should be treated by aspiration.
    (c) Most commonly lies over the occipital bone.
    (d) Does not vary in tension with crying.
    (e) May result in ossification and asymmetry of the skull.

157 (a) **True**
    (b) **True**
    (c) **False**
    (d) **True**   **OB 256**
    (e) **True**

158 (a) **True**
    (b) **False**   Puerperal sepsis is now an infrequent cause of maternal mortality.
    (c) **False**   The source of infection is likely to be from attendants.
                                                                                        OB 257–258
    (d) **False**   This occurs in clostridial infection.
    (e) **False**   Penicillin is the treatment of choice.

159 (a) **False**   There is too much protein in cows' milk.
    (b) **True**
    (c) **True**   Cause and effect are unproven.
    (d) **True**   Cows' milk protein is a powerful antigenic stimulus.
                                                                                        OB 245–248
    (e) **False**   If anything, bottle feeds may be given less frequently because larger volumes can be given.

160 (a) **False**   Encouragement of the flow is important.
    (b) **False**   Diuretics are potentially harmful to the baby.
    (c) **True**   This may be the only way to relieve the discomfort.   **OB 250**
    (d) **False**   Firm support is important.
    (e) **True**

161 (a) **False**   *Staphylococcus aureus* is the commonest organism.
    (b) **True**
    (c) **False**   It is always necessary once an abscess has occurred.
                                                                                        OB 260–261
    (d) **False**   It is usually segmental.
    (e) **True**

162 (a) **True**   Depletion of glycogen stores has occurred *in utero*, so frequent feeding is necessary to prevent this complication.
    (b) **True**   The lack of subcutaneous fat impairs heat conservation.
                                                                                        OB 298–318
    (c) **False**   Pre-term babies, not small for dates babies, develop RDS.
    (d) **False**   Pre-term babies are liable to anaemia.
    (e) **False**   Small for dates babies are not especially prone to infection.

163 (a) **False**   It is a subperiosteal haematoma.
    (b) **False**   This may lead to infection.
    (c) **False**   It is usually over the parietal bones.
    (d) **True**   **OB 302–303**
    (e) **True**

164 Perinatal mortality:
  (a) Includes all stillbirths.
  (b) Includes all neonatal deaths in the first month of life.
  (c) Is increased in Social Classes 4 and 5.
  (d) Is higher for mothers aged under 20 than aged over 35.
  (e) Is principally caused by congenital abnormality, prematurity, and rhesus disease.

165 Respiratory distress syndrome (RDS):
  (a) Usually occurs in infants born before the 34th week of gestation.
  (b) Is more common in caesarean section babies.
  (c) Is more common in babies born to diabetic women.
  (d) Leads to cyanosis.
  (e) Is treated by giving 100 per cent oxygen.

166 Requirements for a newborn baby include:
  (a) 150ml of fluid per kg body weight per 24 hours.
  (b) 110 calories per kg body weight per 24 hours.
  (c) A twice daily bath.
  (d) In breast fed babies, 20 minutes from each breast at each feed.
  (e) 400 IU vitamin D per day.

167 The following are thought to protect against hyaline membrane disease in the neonate:
  (a) Intra-uterine growth retardation.
  (b) Severe pre-eclampsia.
  (c) Heroin addiction.
  (d) Prolonged rupture of the membranes.
  (e) Diabetes.

168 To avoid potential medico-legal problems in breech delivery:
  (a) All breeches should be delivered by Caesarean section.
  (b) The parents should be given the choice of mode of delivery.
  (c) Ultrasound assessment of fetal size should be done.
  (d) X-ray pelvimetry is advisable.
  (e) An epidural anaesthetic should be used.

169 Home confinement is a potential source of litigation because:
  (a) There are inadequate facilities.
  (b) There are unskilled attendants.
  (c) Doctors are reluctant to attend such a confinement.
  (d) There may be delay in obtaining skilled medical help.
  (e) No mechanism exists for proper selection of cases.

164 (a) **True**
   (b) **False** It includes neonatal deaths in the first week of life.
   (c) **True** **OB 344–348**
   (d) **False** Both groups have an increased risk of perinatal mortality, but the over 35s have a higher rate than the under 20s.
   (e) **False** Congenital abnormality, prematurity and *hypoxia* are the causes accounting for 75 per cent of perinatal deaths. Rhesus disease is now a rare cause.

165 (a) **True** After 34 weeks, the fetal lung is generally mature.
   (b) **False** Provided the baby is not pre-term, caesarean section does not predispose to this condition. **OB 316–317**
   (c) **True**
   (d) **True** This is due to shunting of blood through unventilated areas.
   (e) **False** Oxygen concentration should be kept to a minimum necessary to relieve cyanosis.

166 (a) **True**
   (b) **False** 110 calories per kg body weight is all that is required.
   (c) **False** Too frequent bathing may remove the natural skin oils.
OB 300–301
   (d) **False** Ten minutes is usually suficient.
   (e) **True** Breast milk contatins sufficient vitamin D, but artificial feeds may need addition of vitamin D.

167 (a) **True**
   (b) **True** These conditions all stress the fetus and promote surfactant
   (c) **True** production. **OB 316–317**
   (d) **True**
   (e) **False** Surfactant production – in particular the important phosphatidylglycerol component – is retarded in this condition.

168 (a) **False** Litigation may arise from Caesarean section and its complications just as readily as from vaginal delivery.
   (b) **False** Explanation and information should be given to the patient, but a recommendation of mode of delivery should be given.
   (c) **True** Vaginal delivery of very large and very small breech babies is more hazardous so the size should be assessed. **OB 335**
   (d) **True**
   (e) **False** Although there are advantages in good pain relief in the first stage of labour, these may be offset by the loss of bearing down sensation in the second stage.

169 (a) **False** Only low risk cases should be booked for home confinement.
   (b) **False** Health Authorities have a statutory requirement to make available fully qualified midwives for the care of home confinements.
   (c) **False** General practitioners have a statutory duty to attend if called, and most Districts have an Obstetric Flying Squad available to go out in an emergency. **OB 336–337**
   (d) **True** The time factor may be crucial in dealing with an emergency at home.
   (e) **False** General practitioners may advise on the suitability of a case for home confinement, and may refer to a consultant for his opinion.

© 1991 Marcus E Setchell and Richard J Lilford

First published in Great Britain 1985.
Second edition published 1991.

British Library Cataloguing in Publication Data

Setchell, M.
  Multiple choice questions in gynaecology and obstetrics. - 2nd ed.
  I. Title   II. Lilford, R. J.
  618.076

  ISBN 0-340-53710-8

Typeset in Helvetica Light by Hewer Text Compositions Services, Edinburgh.
Printed and bound in Great Britain by Clays Ltd, St. Ives plc for Edward Arnold, a division of Hodder and Stoughton Limited, Mill Road, Dunton Green, Sevenoaks, Kent TN13 2YA.